Cognitive Behavioural Therapy (CBT) for Managing Non-cardiac Chest Pain

CBT for Managing Non-cardiac Chest Pain is an evidence-based guide and workbook for clinicians working with people with non-cardiac chest pain (NCCP). NCCP affects around 25–30% of people in the UK, the US and Europe, and it is associated with high levels of health-care use and compromised quality of life. This is the first book to describe a treatment programme to fill the gap in care for patients.

The authors have developed and researched a novel approach that demonstrates how physiological, cognitive, behavioural and social factors all contribute to the negative experience of chest pain. With the help of exercises and handouts for the patient, the book aims to provide the necessary information and clinical skills and approaches for clinicians to use in health-care settings.

CBT for Managing Non-cardiac Chest Pain will appeal to anyone involved in the care of patients with NCCP, including nurses, general practitioners, cardiologists, acute medical physicians and psychologists.

Elizabeth Marks is a Chartered Clinical Psychologist and accredited CBT Practitioner. She works at University College London Hospital and is a Lecturer in Clinical Psychology at the University of Bath. Elizabeth's particular interests lie in enabling people to better manage chronic illness and to reduce the emotional, physical and functional consequences of physical health problems, such as chest pain. She has published a number of articles on non-cardiac chest pain.

Myra Hunter is Emeritus Professor of clinical health psychology with King's College London. She has specialized in the application of psychology to cardiology, oncology and women's health and has published over 200 articles and chapters and 7 books. Her clinical research has focused on developing interventions to help people manage persistent physical symptoms such as chest pain.

John Chambers is Professor of Clinical Cardiology and consultant cardiologist at Guy's and St Thomas' Hospitals, London. He has a career-long interest in the interactions between physical and psychological processes in non-cardiac chest pain. John has published 8 books and over 300 papers on general medicine, heart valve disease, chest pain and cardiac imaging.

Non-cardiac chest pain affects as many as 80% of patients attending chest pain clinics yet treatment is suboptimal. These patients have been consistently shown to continue to report symptoms and functional impairments and to be high users of expensive health care. This timely book addresses this neglected public health problem, and provides clear account of assessment and management. The authors have adopted a multidisciplinary, "stepped care" approach to treatment which has been shown to be effective in reducing chest pain frequency as well as improving behaviour and well being. The book deserves to be widely read by practitioners working in both primary and tertiary care settings. GPs, emergency room clinicians and cardiologists will find it particularly useful.

—Christopher Bass, *Consultant in Liaison Psychiatry*
John Radcliffe Hospital

CBT for Managing Non-cardiac Chest Pain

- An Evidence-based Guide

Elizabeth Marks, Myra Hunter and John Chambers

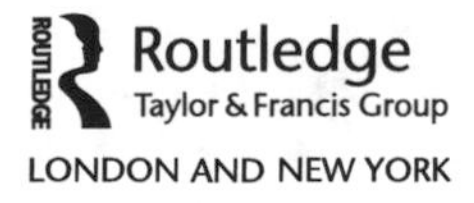
LONDON AND NEW YORK

First published 2017
by Routledge
2 Park Square, Milton Park, Abingdon, Oxon OX14 4RN

and by Routledge
711 Third Avenue, New York, NY 10017

Routledge is an imprint of the Taylor & Francis Group, an informa business

British Library Cataloguing-in-Publication Data
A catalogue record for this book is available from the British Library

Library of Congress Cataloging-in-Publication Data
Names: Marks, Elizabeth, 1981– author. | Hunter, Myra, author. | Chambers, John (John Boyd), author.
Title: CBT for managing non-cardiac chest pain : an evidence-based guide / Elizabeth Marks, Myra Hunter and John Chambers.
Description: Abingdon, Oxon ; New York, NY : Routledge, 2017. | Includes bibliographical references.
Identifiers: LCCN 2016022878 | ISBN 9781138119000 (hardback) | ISBN 9781138119017 (pbk.) | ISBN 9781315629254 (ebook)
Subjects: | MESH: Chest Pain—therapy | Cognitive Therapy—methods | Evidence-Based Medicine—methods
Classification: LCC RC489.C63 | NLM WF 970 | DDC 616.89/1425—dc23
LC record available at https://lccn.loc.gov/2016022878

ISBN: 978-1-138-11900-0 (hbk)
ISBN: 978-1-138-11901-7 (pbk)
ISBN: 978-1-315-62925-4 (ebk)

Typeset in Stone Serif
by Apex CoVantage, LLC

Contents

Figures

Tables

Acknowledgements

We would like to thank Victoria Russell, Lisa Knisely and Leoni Bryan for their input to the running of our multidisciplinary clinic, and to the men and women who attended the clinic and from whom we learnt so much.

We would also like to thank Phillip Bentley of National Services for Health Improvement (NSHI) for doing the graphic design.

Section 1

Non-cardiac chest pain and biopsychosocial approaches

Introduction

Why is this book needed?

Chest pain is common. It is usually distressing because of its association with heart disease, and it can become chronic if untreated (Marks et al., 2014). However, chest pain is most frequently benign. Non-cardiac causes are approximately four times more common than coronary disease or other dangerous conditions. Understandably, because missing coronary disease can lead to myocardial infarction or death, the main focus is on detecting coronary disease. There are detailed protocols to enable health professionals to do this that were drawn up by professional bodies, including the European Cardiac Society and the American Heart Association (Gibbons et al., 2007; Montalescot et al., 2013).

Once coronary disease has been excluded, the modern medical management process typically runs out of momentum. There are no international guidelines to manage non-cardiac chest pain (NCCP). Patients with NCCP generally remain unassured by negative cardiac investigations and have a high level of pain and psychological distress (Chambers et al., 2013; Marks et al., 2014), high unemployment rates and heavy use of health-care resources (Eslick and Talley, 2004; Fagring et al., 2010; Christoph et al., 2014). The causation and maintenance of NCCP may be complex given the interaction of organic and psychological processes. However, treatment can be effectively delivered at a relatively low cost. In this book, we aim to describe a biopsychosocial approach that can be used to understand NCCP and help patients manage it.

A biopsychosocial approach

Health emerges from an interactive network of biological, psychological and social factors. The cause and maintenance of NCCP often involves a complex interaction of organic and psychological processes (Chambers et al., 2013). To fully understand each individual with NCCP, all of these factors must be considered. This requires a full medical assessment to identify any organic factors and a thorough psychosocial assessment to identify the cognitive, emotional, behavioural and social influences on pain. An alternative biopsychosocial explanation can then be developed with an individualized treatment plan. This may include an effective medical or physical treatment, as well as specific psychological management strategies.

Once heart disease has been excluded, it is possible to identify alternative physical causes (such as gastro-oesophageal reflux or musculoskeletal disorder). There may be psychological factors influencing NCCP (such as anxiety, behavioural changes and fearful beliefs about the meaning of chest pain) and important social and lifestyle factors (such as stressful life events and the responses of other people, including health-care professionals). These factors can influence and exacerbate chest pain in a vicious cycle (see Figure I.1), which explains how and why NCCP persists. We explore these various factors in more detail in Chapter 4.

This book offers an overview of the epidemiology of NCCP, followed by an explanation of how to assess patients with NCCP. It then offers a treatment strategy based on cognitive behavioural therapy (CBT) that identifies potential solutions and effective coping strategies for NCCP. CBT has been identified as the most effective and reliable treatment for NCCP in recent Cochrane Reviews (Kisely et al., 2010; 2012). Studies have found that an important part of successful treatment is an initial, comprehensive and therapeutic assessment. This involves investigation of the multiple factors affecting chest pain followed by unambiguous reassurance and written information (Mayou et al., 1999). Of those patients who remain distressed, many can benefit from further support using 'low-intensity' CBT delivered in the format of guided self-help, whilst others may require a 'high-intensity' CBT intervention in the context of extreme distress or complicating factors (Chambers et al., 2014).

This book is based on our biopsychosocial chest pain clinic run by a cardiologist, cardiac nurses and psychologists. It has been found to

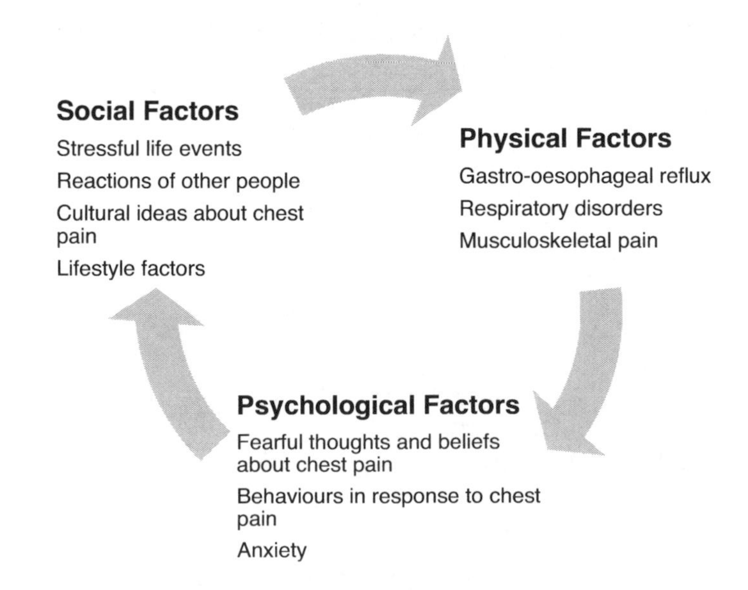

Figure I.1 The biopsychosocial model of chest pain indicating the types of biological, psychological and social factors that may be important in NCCP.

lead to significant benefits for many people with persistent chest pain (Chambers et al., 2014; Marks et al., 2016). The clinic team developed this book as an evidence-based guide based on their experiences and knowledge of working with chest pain. It can be used by a range of health-care professionals working with people who have NCCP, such as cardiologists, nurses, psychologists, CBT therapists, psychological well-being practitioners and general practitioners.

Chapter 1 begins by offering an overview of NCCP and its prevalence, prognosis and impact on people's quality of life. In Chapter 2, we describe how to differentiate NCCP from chest pain caused by cardiac disease. It is important that coronary artery disease is excluded before you and the person with chest pain feel confident in engaging in this treatment approach. Chapter 3 offers an overview of the historical and sociocultural perspectives of chest pain and how these shape a person's reactions to NCCP. In Chapter 4, we look at biopsychosocial approaches to pain in general, and in Chapter 5 we look at the biological and psychosocial factors specific to NCCP. Chapter 6 provides an overview of CBT and how this is used within a biopsychosocial approach to NCCP. In Chapter 7 we draw this information together in a way that will support the clinician in conducting comprehensive, therapeutic assessments. This includes a structured assessment protocol.

The second part of the book is a workbook that guides treatment. It gives detailed information to allow the treating clinician to provide guided self-help (sometimes known as low-intensity CBT) to patients with persistent NCCP. This workbook does not train the clinician to become a CBT practitioner and does not qualify them to deliver standard (or high intensity) CBT. Rather, as seen in other forms of 'low intensity' CBT, it offers a standardized intervention grounded in CBT principles that includes a variety of strategies known to be helpful in NCCP. It is appropriate for delivery by a clinician who has had some training in CBT preferably closely supervised by a CBT practitioner. For example, delivery by a cardiac nurse who has completed a short training in the basics of CBT and who with their CBT supervisor regularly. The treating clinician should follow the workbook closely, session by session, taking any issues not covered by the manual to the supervising CBT specialist. The workbook includes handouts and audio resources for the patient, and all of these are available in the appendices or can be downloaded at www.routledge.com/9781138119017. In the third part of the book, there is a list of other resources that may support the clinician in this work and which may also be of use to patients.

All of the information in this book is based on our biopsychosocial chest pain clinic, which has already helped many people struggling with NCCP. We hope that the ideas and strategies suggested in the book will offer similar support and help to other people who continue to struggle with this chronic and disabling condition and to the clinicians working with them.

References

Chambers, J.B., Marks, E.M., Knisley, L., & Hunter, M. (2013). Non-cardiac chest pain: Time to extend the rapid access chest pain clinic? *Int J Clin Pract* 67: 303–6.

Chambers, J.B., Marks, E.M., Russell, V., & Hunter, M.S. (2014). A multidisciplinary, biopsychosocial treatment for non-cardiac chest pain. *Int J Clin Practice* 69(9): 922–7. doi:10.1111/ijcp.12533

Christoph, M., Christoph, A., Dannemmann, S., Poitz, D., Pfluecke, C., Strasser, R.H., Wunderlich, C., Koellner, V., & Ibrahim, K. (2014). Mental symptoms in patients with cardiac symptoms and normal coronary arteries. *Openheart* 1: e000093. doi:10.1136/openrt-2014-000093.

Eslick, G.D., & Talley, N.J. (2004). Non-cardiac chest pain: Predictors of health care seeking, the types of health care professional consulted, work absenteeism and interruption of daily activities. *Aliment Pharmacol Ther* 20: 909–15.

Fagring, A.J., Lappas, G., Kjellgren, K.I., Welin, C., Manhem, K., & Rosengren, A. (2010). Twenty-year trends in incidence and 1-year mortality in Swedish patients hospitalised with non-AMI chest pain. Data from 1987–2006 from the Swedish hospital and death registries. *Heart* 96: 1043–9.

Gibbons, R.J., Abrams, J., & Chatterjee, K. et al. (2007). Chronic angina focused update of the ACC/AHA 2002 guidelines for the management of patients with chronic stable angina: A report of the American College of Cardiology/American Heart Association Task Force on Practice Guidelines Writing Group to develop the focused update of the 2002 guidelines for the management of patients with chronic stable angina. *Circulation* 116: 2762–72.

Kisley, S.R., Campbell, L.A., Yelland, M.J., & Paydar, A. (2012). Psychological interventions for symptomatic management of non-specific chest pain in patients with normal coronary anatomy. *Cochrane Database Systematic Review* 13(6).

Marks, E.M., Chambers, J.B., Russell, V., & Hunter, M.S. (2014). The rapid access chest pain clinic: Unmet distress and disability. Q J Med 107(6): 429–34.

Marks, E.M., Chambers, J.B., Russell, V., & Hunter, M.S. (2016). A novel cognitive behavioural stepped-care intervention for patients with non-cardiac chest pain. *Health Psychol Behav Med* 4(1): 15–28.

Mayou, R.A., Bass, C.M., & Bryant, B.M. (1999). Management of non-cardiac chest pain: From research to clinical practice. *Heart* 81(4): 387–92.

Montalescot, G., Sechtem, U., Achenbach, S., Andreotti, F., Arden, C., Budaj, A., Bugiardini, R., Crea, F., Cuisset, T., Di Mario, C., & Ferreira, J.R. (2013). ESC guidelines on the management of stable coronary artery disease: The task force on the management of stable coronary artery disease of the European Society of Cardiology. *Europ Heart J* 34: 2949–3003.

Chapter 1

What is non-cardiac chest pain?

Chest pain is an almost universal experience. Most people have experienced chest pain at times without being concerned by it. However, people seek advice for a variety of reasons, such as if they have severe or recurrent pain, a family history of coronary disease, anxiety about health in general or concerns as a result of health-care advertisements or public health campaigns (Figure 1.1). The prime reason for help-seeking tends to be an understandable concern, or in many cases fear, that the pain signifies a threat to health, typically a heart attack. In some cases, the general practitioner (GP) may be confident to reassure the person that the pain is benign without performing tests. Otherwise the patient might be referred to a specialist, usually to a cardiologist or to a rapid access chest pain clinic (RACPC), or less commonly to a gastroenterologist, rheumatologist or psychologist.

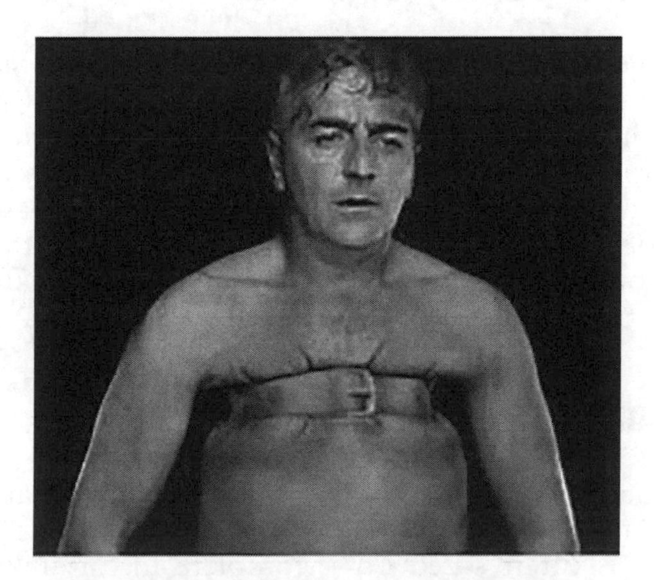

Figure 1.1 Image used in the poster for the British Heart Foundation 2006 doubt kills campaign. The caption read 'A chest pain is your body saying call 999'.

Source: Reproduced with the kind permission of TBWA/London.

Someone referred to a cardiac service with chest pain is likely to have tests to rule out coronary disease (see Chapter 2). If the test results are normal, the pain is likely to be labelled non-cardiac chest pain (NCCP), and further investigation of alternative possible mechanisms for the pain are not routinely performed. For ease of communication we use the term NCCP throughout the book. NCCP is a label that tends to be offered after the exclusion of coronary disease. It is not a unitary diagnosis. Nonetheless, there are sufficient features common to patients with this label of exclusion to describe an epidemiology and natural history.

How common is non-cardiac chest pain?

The lifetime population prevalence of NCCP is approximately 20–33% (Fass and Achem, 2011; Chambers et al., 2015) compared with approximately 6–7% for angina across the globe. The incidence of NCCP depends on the clinical setting. It is found in 70–80% of patients presenting to a GP with chest pain or referred by a GP to a RACPC (Sekhri et al., 2007). These are usually patients with chronic stable pain. For those presenting with acute onset chest pain to an emergency department, the incidence of NCCP is approximately 50% (Blatchford and Capewell, 1999). Coronary angiography is performed diagnostically in some patients admitted with acute chest pain even without abnormalities of the ECG or cardiac biomarkers. It may also be performed in patients with persistent chronic chest pain. Normal coronary anatomy, implying NCCP, is found in 40% having diagnostic coronary angiography (Patel et al., 2010).

Characteristics of a patient with NCCP

The average age is in the late 40s, and males and females are equally represented (Chambers et al., 2015). About one-third have cardiac risk factors. The majority have pain that is atypical of a cardiac origin (see next section). Symptoms from overbreathing, tension headache and bowel motility disorders are commonly associated with the pain (Table 1.1). Anxiety and depression are as common as in patients with proven coronary disease, but they tend not to resolve and are associated with more negative or extreme illness beliefs (Chambers et al., 2015).

What is the pain like?

About one-quarter of patients report chest pain 'typical' of a cardiac origin, meaning that it is precipitated by exertion and relieved by rest. However, this is often based on incomplete history-taking, as many patients have pain at variable times. For example, it may be occasionally rather than reproducibly related to exertion. If related to exercise, it may develop after rather than during exercise, or the chest pain may last

Table 1.1 Vignette of a characteristic patient with NCCP

Male or female in the late 40s
Mild heavy feeling across the chest all the time
Additional 'jabs' of pain at a variable site most commonly around the left breast area; may radiate to left shoulder or arm
Pain can come at any time including rest or minimal exertion; may last for hours after exercise
Palpitation with the pain or at other times
Irritable bowel (abdominal pain and bloating, flatulence, variable stool consistency, urgency)
Headaches, fatigue, 'muzzy' head, difficulty concentrating
Cannot take a satisfying breath
Sighing thoracic respiratory pattern, frequent throat clearing
Breath-holding time reduced to less than 20 seconds
Pain reproduced by chest wall palpation or by breath-holding
Stresses in life
Thinks he or she may have a heart attack
Frequently off work

Source: Modified from Chambers et al., 2015, with kind permission from BMJ publishing.

for hours or even days after exercise. Sometimes the pain is triggered by trivial exercise. All these features are uncharacteristic of coronary disease despite there initially being an apparent relationship to exercise. It is easy, but potentially unhelpful, to over-report typicality in an effort to avoid missing coronary disease. In one study (Day and Sowton, 1976), 60% of patients with normal coronary angiography had pain occasionally related to exercise, but only 16% had pain reproducibly precipitated by exercise. The proportion with truly typical pain was therefore 16% rather than 60%. The subjectivity of the history is underlined by a study (Faxon et al., 1982) in which 45% were initially thought to have 'atypical' pain. This figure rose to 80% when the history was retaken after the finding of normal coronary anatomy at coronary angiography.

To try to improve the objectivity of the history, we compared chest pain characteristics in 65 patients with completely normal coronary anatomy (i.e. cardiac pain effectively excluded) and 65 with proven coronary disease (Cooke et al., 1997). We used 50 questions, including some modified from the Rose Questionnaire (Rose et al., 1977; Bass et al., 1989; Fischbacher et al., 2001), which is commonly used for epidemiological studies. Three of the 50 questions allowed a statistical differentiation of patients with normal and diseased coronary arteries (Table 1.2). These were also the clinically obvious questions since they explored the occurrence of the pain with exercise or rest and its duration. The advantage of the statistical treatment is that it gave more precise numbers out of 10 to suggest whether an answer was typical or atypical. This then allowed a typicality score to be derived: 0 (non-cardiac pain), 1 or 2 (atypical pain), or 3 (typical pain). This scoring system was shown to predict coronary disease or its absence better than treadmill exercise testing in an

Table 1.2 The Guy's Chest Pain Questionnaire

	Score 1 if the answer is	*Score 0 if the answer is*
1 If you have 10 pains (or tightness or breathlessness) in a row, how many occur on exercise?	10	0–9
2 How many occur at rest?	0–1	2–10
3 How long does the pain last?	≤5 min	>5 min

These questions are asked, and the questionnaire is scored to give a total of the three questions. Scoring is as follows:

0 = Non-cardiac pain
1 or 2 = atypical pain
3 = typical pain

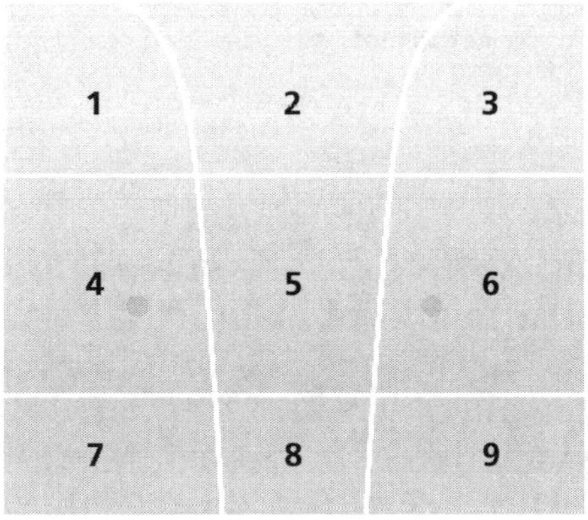

	Normal n = 65	Abnormal n = 65	OR
1	5 (8%)	3 (5%)	1.72
2	11 (17%)	16 (25%)	0.62
3	11 (17%)	13 (20%)	0.81
4	23 (35%)	10 (15%)	3.01*
5	55 (85%)	41 (63%)	3.22†
6	38 (58%)	18 (28%)	3.67‡
7	7 (11%)	3 (5%)	2.49
8	10 (15%)	7 (11%)	1.51
9	10 (15%)	3 (5%)	3.76

*$P<0.05$ †$P<0.01$ ‡$P<0.001$

Figure 1.2 Distribution of chest pain in 65 patients with normal coronary arteries and 65 with diseased coronary arteries. The left panel shows a diagram of the chest wall with sectors marked out and numbered. We asked 65 people with proven coronary disease (abnormal) and 65 people with NCCP and normal coronary arteries (normal) where they experienced their pain. The frequency with which each sector was named is shown in the table on the right with percentages of the total in parentheses. The odds ratio (OR) is shown in the far right column with an assessment of statistical significance for the difference between people with normal and abnormal coronary arteries. The figure shows that people with NCCP were more likely than those with angina from coronary disease to experience chest pain in sectors 4, 5 or 6, most commonly in the central sector, 5.

Source: Reproduced by permission of BMJ publishers from Cooke et al. (1997).

outpatient population (Wu et al., 2001). Patients with normal coronary arteries were more likely to experience pain in the axilla on the left more than the right (Figure 1.2). Surprisingly, although both groups had pain in the middle of the chest, which is textbook for cardiac pain, this was actually statistically more common for patients with normal (85%) than abnormal (63%) ($p < 0.01$) coronary arteries. There were no differences in the radiation of the pain or in the quality (gripping, stabbing, burning) between the two groups. This is an important observation because lay and medical texts often differentiate cardiac and non-cardiac pain from these qualitative features.

Another important observation was that a similar proportion of people with normal (71%) and abnormal coronary arteries (74%) reported that sublingual glyceryl trinitrate (GTN) improved their pain. This response is often, incorrectly, thought to be characteristic of cardiac pain. However, patients with abnormal coronary arteries were statistically more likely to find that GTN abolished chest pain quickly, while patients with normal coronary arteries tended to report that the pain only reduced after more than 5 minutes, which is not compatible with its pharmacological action.

One mechanism of NCCP is an abnormal thoracic, as opposed to a normal abdominal, breathing pattern. The pain is variable and may occur at rest, with minimal exertion and commonly at any time. There is often a sensation of fullness or heaviness which may be present all the time and a brassiere or shirt may become uncomfortable. Overbreathing is associated with a feeling of 'air hunger' – being unable to fill the lungs properly or take a satisfying breath. The patient may react with deep breathing, which makes it worse. There may be throat-clearing and a sensation of globus ('something stuck in the throat'). Breathlessness during eating or talking (for example, on the telephone) is common. There may be a 'pins and needles' feeling around the mouth or the fingers usu ally on the left and occasionally sensitivity to noise or light. A muzzy head or inability to concentrate is common.

Oesophageal pain may sometimes occur with exercise, but it is much more likely to be precipitated by large meals or acidic or fatty foods and by bending or lying down. It may be improved by antacids. Other oesophageal symptoms may be present including heartburn, acid reflux into the mouth (water brash) and occasional regurgitation of food. Heartburn can also occur with irritable bowel syndrome. Dysphagia is specific for an oesophageal abnormality, but it is uncommon.

Musculoskeletal pain may also be precipitated by exercise but usually when this includes movement of the arms, back or the affected joint. The pain from carpal tunnel syndrome sometimes radiates to the left side of the chest. There may be localized tenderness, although, surprisingly, this did not differentiate our patients with and without proven coronary disease (Cooke et al., 1997).

The natural history of NCCP

Cardiologists consider NCCP as benign because the incidence of myocardial infarction or premature death is close to zero (Chambers and Bass, 1990; Fagring et al., 2010). Yet patients remain significantly disabled, reporting high levels of distress, impaired quality of life and work absenteeism (Robertson et al., 2008; Parkash et al., 2009).

About three-quarters report residual chest pain and continue seeing a physician. One-half remain or become unemployed and absenteeism is common with a mean time off work of 22 days (range 1–240) in a year. Health care use is high. In the 6 months before coming to our clinic (Chambers et al., 2014), 63% of referrals saw a GP three or more times, 63% saw a cardiologist three or more times, 33% saw another hospital doctor and 28% attended the emergency room more than once. In the USA in 1989, it was estimated that bed costs alone were $3,500 in the year after a normal coronary angiogram (Richter et al., 1989).

Persistence of chest pain is strongly related to biopsychosocial factors. Symptoms are likely to continue if an underlying organic non-cardiac source of pain or psychological factors, such as health anxiety, are not addressed (Chambers et al., 2015). There are strong associations between NCCP and stress at home or work and negative life events. A number of psychological processes have been identified in the maintenance of NCCP, including catastrophizing, avoidance behaviour and a belief that the heart is the source of the pain and that symptoms are uncontrollable. Chronicity may also be associated with a longer interval before diagnosis potentially because this leads to long-term changes in the individual's behaviour and social world, for example, receiving a disability allowance, using a wheelchair or being prescribed domiciliary oxygen. We conducted a study exploring the levels of distress and disability of patients with cardiac versus non-cardiac chest pain, finding the two groups comparable on many outcomes (Box 1.1).

BOX 1.1 DISTRESS AND DISABILITY IN THE CHEST PAIN CLINIC (MARKS ET AL., 2014)

We compared the characteristics of patients with cardiac chest pain (CCP) versus non-cardiac chest pain (NCCP) attending a rapid access chest pain clinic in a large urban hospital over an 18-month period. Patients completed a number of questionnaires and cross-sectional comparisons were made on measures of mood, beliefs, somatic symptoms and health-care use.

We found that there were no significant differences between the two groups of patients in terms of their chest pain (frequency, severity, duration or related distress). Levels of anxiety and depression were also equivalent between groups, and both had similar levels of health-care use, although NCCP patients reported seeing more types of health-care workers. Both groups reported equivalent levels of impairment in work and social functioning and a restriction of exercise because of cardiac-related concerns. There were some differences, with the NCCP group being younger on average and reporting more atypical pain. They also reported higher levels of panic-type beliefs about chest pain and reported less illness coherence (indicating that they made less sense of their chest pain). Overall, this study demonstrated that NCCP is as distressing and disabling as cardiac pain.

Descriptions of chest pain given by patients with NCCP

Patients attending the RACPC and our biopsychosocial treatment clinic report a huge variation in the type, frequency and location of pain (Box 1.2).

BOX 1.2 DESCRIPTIONS OF CHEST PAIN FROM PATIENTS ATTENDING OUR CLINIC

Exertional pain: *"The pain is getting worse. It comes whenever I am rushing, and makes me so tired, I just don't want to be active any more. I feel really scared, so I have to sit still until it goes."*

"I get chest pain mostly when I'm rushing somewhere, so I've stopped playing sports."

"The heart test (stress echo) was really scary and my heart pounded hard and I felt weak afterwards."

Pain occurring at any time: *"I get the pain whenever and it can last for minutes or hours. Nothing helps. Sometimes I'm short of breath but I put it down to stress."*

"It happens any time. It makes me sweat, shake and have blurred vision so it must be serious."

Constant pain: *"Chest pain is there all of the time, but it gets sharper sometimes. It feels a bit better if I move my arm or take paracetamol."*

"When I get chest pain, I don't feel well and look pale in the mirror. I have the pain all the time except for 5 minutes after I wake up. I panic when I think that I will die like my mum and uncles."

Thoracic breathing: *"I get the pain when I'm rushing or stressed. It's a stabbing in my chest. I get a dry mouth and can't breathe properly, like I'm being strangled. It can happen at any time."*

Oesophageal pain: *"I get burning in my chest. I've always had reflux and drinking water helps. But it's getting worse and now it happens when I lie down and I feel breathless."*

"I have acid in my mouth and I get stomach pain a lot. I have a sore back too. Chest pain comes out of the blue, I can't stop it."

"The first time was at Christmas when I ate too much. I have IBS which also affects me badly."

Musculoskeletal pain: *"I get a burning in my chest and can't breathe. The pain is all down the left side of my body and my arm is numb. It lasts all day, and it happens most days."*

"I get an 'electric' pain down my arm which leads to my heart. It feels like a muscle stops in my heart. It's on the left so can't be from my skeleton. Rubbing it can help, but nothing else does."

"I get sensations in my heart sometimes. I've had pain in my back and chest since I had my kids. Codydramol can help a bit."

"My first episode of chest pain felt like burning in my chest and arm. My chest is sore to touch."

"I get chest pain when I bend over or do DIY so I don't do much exercise any more. I've had back pain for years, but it feels completely different."

Different types of pain: *"I've had four or five episodes of violent pain, with milder pain in between. I think the milder pains are muscular, but the severe ones feel dangerous."*

"I have three pains: one comes and goes and is okay, one is bothersome and affects my breathing every few days and the third is rarer but scary, like an electric shock, which stops me in my tracks."

Few patients reaching such services will have had the non-cardiac, organic causes of chest pain either identified or treated. Many may need intervention in the form of medication for gastro-oesophageal reflux, asthma or neuropathic pain, referral to a physiotherapist or even simple advice. For example, one patient described muscular pain down the left side of his body, and he explained how he had changed his sleeping position since developing glaucoma in his left eye. He disliked going to bed if he could not see the room and therefore had to sleep with the right hip upwards, lying on his left side. This led to increased pressure and muscle pain on his left. A simple explanation and a change in his sleeping position cured the problem.

High levels of psychological distress are reported by many patients with chest pain. Sometimes this indicates untreated psychiatric or psychological disorders requiring further support from local mental health services, such as health anxiety:

> *It's not just the pain, but I have flu symptoms that keep coming back and they've made my muscles funny. I can't go to the gym because I get so tired. I lost my appetite too. I felt better for a short while, after the GP reassured me about my symptoms. I'm seeing an ENT specialist now, because I had a sore throat. They found a node on my thyroid but told me not to worry, but of course I'm worried! I get pins and needles in my hands and worry this means there is something wrong. I often get anxious about small things. I don't like talking about my health, but I do check things on the Internet a lot.*

High levels of depression, anxiety and panic are frequently described:

> *My husband died last year and now his parents are contesting custody of our children. I'm really stressed and get panic attacks where I feel very tense and get palpitations. I'm fed up and find it difficult to cope. Sometimes I think about ending it all, but I keep going because of my children.*

Stress and difficult life events are very common in people attending the biopsychosocial NCCP clinic. In some cases, it is possible to identify stress as a trigger for the first episode of chest pain:

> *The first time I had chest pain was about six months ago . . . I had just lost my job and was worried about how I could support my family. The year before that my partner was diagnosed with cancer. It has been really stressful and at the time I was eating more, worrying all the time and couldn't relax at all.*

In other cases, it is possible to identify ongoing stress as a potential factor in NCCP persistence. This may not always be recognized by the individual as a relevant factor:

> *Lots of people at work are getting laid off. I would like to move to offices closer to home because at the moment I'm commuting for four hours a*

day. I never used to worry but now I worry all the time. I'm exhausted. I don't know what I'll do if I lose my job.

Other people report a clear link between feeling stressed and chest pain:

Since my normal test results I think chest pain must be stress related and, when I think about it, I never have chest pain when I'm on holiday. I'm still perplexed though because no one has told me what the cause is.

The relevant psychosocial processes (thoughts, feelings and behaviours) usually become clear when speaking to people about their chest pain. A very common belief is that chest pain is a sign of a heart attack. This often relates to experiences of friends or family with heart problems. There is also a lot of publicity about seeking medical help for chest pain, including a poster campaign by the British Heart Foundation in 2006 stressing the possible dangers from chest pain caused by coronary disease (see Figure 1.1). There are common themes about not knowing what NCCP actually is and being unable to control it.

My brother died from a heart attack 15 years ago, he was only 49. I'm scared it will happen to me too. The tests are not reassuring because I still haven't been given a reason for the pain.

I'm worried that I've damaged my heart as I used to be an alcoholic and my friend has just been told he has cardiomyopathy from alcohol.

Chest pain just comes out of the blue, I don't know why and there is nothing I can do to stop it.

The hospital told me my heart was okay, but then what is going on? Perhaps it is cancer or a problem with my muscles? I really don't know.

A large number of people with NCCP describe major life changes subsequent to chest pain:

I've had chest pain for 2 years. It means that I've stopped going to the gym, stopped working, playing with my daughter, running – everything really. The first episode happened at the train station and I had to get an ambulance to the hospital. I still don't know what it is, it must be a serious heart problem.

It's affected my life so much because it is all I can think about.

I'm down because I'm not working. The doctor told me to stop at first, but now he says I'm fit to work again. It doesn't feel like that to me. I can't do most of the things I used to do, and I'm scared about what might happen if I start doing them. I monitor my heart all the time in case something happens.

Summary

The proportion of patients with chest pain caused by heart disease is relatively small. Once a cardiac cause is excluded, there are a number of non-cardiac organic causes that should be considered. Additionally, psychosocial factors can cause, contribute to and maintain NCCP. Consequently, there are a large numbers of patients with persistent chest pain from non-cardiac causes that require specialist treatment approaches. Targeting these non-cardiac factors is the focus of our biopsychosocial approach to NCCP. Before describing NCCP and the methods of our clinic in more detail, the next chapter gives an overview of coronary disease and how they can be excluded.

References

Bass, E.B., Follansbee, W.P., & Orchard, T.J. (1989). Comparison of a supplemented Rose questionnaire to exercise thallium testing in men and women. *J Clin Epidemiol* 42: 385–94.

Blatchford, O., & Capewell, S. (1999). Emergency medical admissions in Glasgow: General practices vary despite adjustments for age, sex and deprivation. *Brit J Gen Prac* 49: 551–4.

Chambers, J., & Bass, C. (1990). Chest pain with normal coronary anatomy: A review of natural history and possible etiologic factors. *Prog Cardiovasc Dis* 33: 161–84.

Chambers, J.B., Marks, E.M., & Hunter, M.S. (2015). The head says yes but the heart says no: What is non-cardiac chest pain and how is it managed? *Heart Educ* 101: 1240–9.

Chambers, J.B., Marks, E.M., Russell, V., & Hunter, M.S. (2014). A multidisciplinary, biopsychosocial treatment for non-cardiac chest pain. *Int J Clin Practice* 69(9): 922–7. doi:10.1111/ijcp.12533

Cooke, R., Smeeton, N., & Chambers, J. (1997). Comparative study of chest pain characteristics in patients with normal and abnormal coronary angiograms. *Heart* 78: 142–6.

Day, L.J., & Sowton, E. (1976). Clinical features and follow-up of patients with angina and normal coronary arteries. *Lancet* 2: 334–7.

Fagring, A.J., Lappas, G., Kjellgren, K.I., Welin, C., Manhem, K., & Rosengren, A. (2010). Twenty-year trends in incidence and 1-year mortality in Swedish patients hospitalised with non-AMI chest pain. Data from 1987–2006 from the Swedish hospital and death registries. *Heart* 96: 1043–9.

Fass, R., & Achem, S.R. (2011). Noncardiac chest pain: Epidemiology, natural course and pathogenesis. *J Neurgastroenterol Motil* 17: 110–23.

Faxon, D.P., McCabe, C.H., Kreigel, D.E., & Ryan, T.J. (1982). Therapeutic and economic value of a normal coronary angiogram. *Am J Med* 73: 500–5.

Fischbacher, C.M., Bhopal, R., Unwin, N., White, M., & Alberti, K.G.M.M. (2001). The performance of the Rose angina questionnaire in South

Asian and European origin populations: A comparative study in Newcastle, UK. *Int J Epidemiol* 30: 1009–16.
Marks, E.M., Chambers, J.B., Russell, V., & Hunter, M.S. (2014). The rapid access chest pain clinic: Unmet distress and disability. *Q J Med* 107(6): 429–34.
Parkash, O., Almas, A., Hameed, A., & Islam, M. (2009). Comparison of non cardiac chest pain (NCCP) and acute coronary syndrome (ACS) patients presenting to a tertiary care centre. *J Pak Med Ass* 59: 667–71.
Patel, M.R., Peterson, E.D., Dai, D., Brennan, J.M., Redberg, R.F., Anderson, H.V., Brindis, R.G., & Douglas, P.S. (2010). Low diagnostic yield of elective coronary angiography. *New Engl J Med* 362: 886–95.
Richter, J.E., Bradley, L.A., & Castell, D.O. (1989). Esophageal chest pain: Current controversies in pathogenesis, diagnosis, and therapy. *Ann Int Med* 110: 66–78.
Robertson, N., Javed, N., Samani, N.J., & Khunti, K. (2008). Psychological morbidity and illness appraisals of patients with cardiac and non-cardiac chest pain attending a rapid access chest pain clinic: A longitudinal cohort study. *Heart* 94: e12.
Rose, G., McCartney, P., & Reid, D.D. (1977). Self-administration of a questionnaire on chest pain and intermittent claudication. *Br J Prev Soc Med* 31(1): 42–48.
Sekhri, N., Feder, G.S., Junghans, C., Hemingway, H., & Timmis, A.D. (2007). How effective are rapid access chest pain clinics? Prognosis of incident angina and non-cardiac chest pain in 8762 consecutive patients. *Heart* 93: 458–63.
Wu, E., Smeeton, N., & Chambers, J.B. (2001). A chest pain score for stratifying the risk of coronary artery disease in patients having day-case coronary angiography. *Int J Cardiol* 78: 257–64.

Chapter 2

What is coronary disease and how is it excluded?

Non-cardiac chest pain is usually a diagnosis of exclusion, and this book assumes that cardiac pain has been excluded to a clinically appropriate degree. To clarify the difference between pain of a cardiac origin and NCCP, we will give an overview of coronary disease and how it can be excluded.

What is coronary disease?

There is an underlying abnormality of the endothelium, the inner lining of blood vessels, leading to the development of atheroma in medium and large arteries, including those around the heart. Atheroma consists of cholesterol accumulation associated with inflammation, fibrosis and smooth muscle proliferation. Ultimately calcification may occur. The mechanisms of chronic stable angina and myocardial infarction are different.

Chronic stable angina

Atheroma initially causes no significant encroachment on the inside space of a coronary artery (the lumen), but starts to reduce blood flow on exercise when it reduces the inner diameter by about 70% or more. This causes myocardial ischaemia, a restriction of blood supply to the heart, usually resulting in angina although occasionally in arrhythmia or ischaemic cardiomyopathy (heart muscle disease). The atheroma may affect one, two or all three main coronary arteries (Figure 2.1). Luckily the coronary circulation has adaptive mechanisms to protect itself against blockage. The coronary circulation consists of an array of progressively smaller branches off the three main arteries culminating in a network of arterioles and capillaries. In response to repetitive ischaemia, collateral vessels develop around the developing coronary stenosis resulting in effectively a spontaneous 'internal bypass' with protective results similar to those of surgical grafting. This means that there may be no ischaemia despite a severe anatomical lesion on a contrast angiography, and a heart attack may not develop even if the vessel becomes completely blocked.

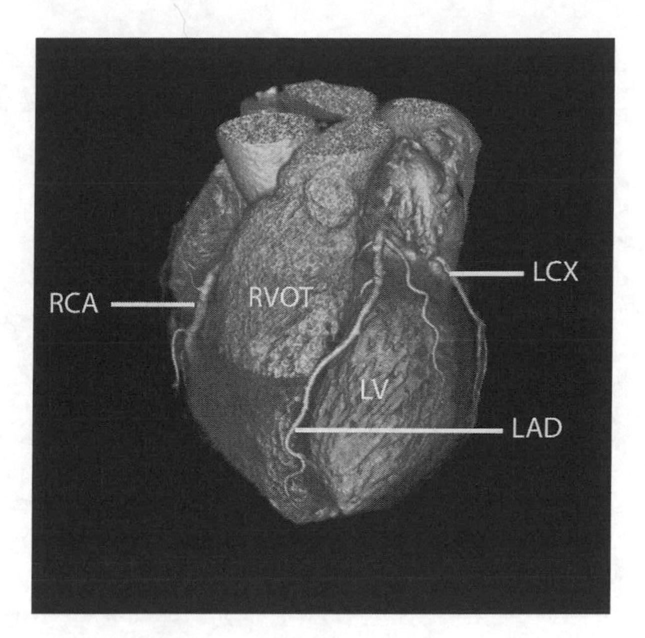

Figure 2.1 3-D reconstructed CT scan showing the coronary anatomy

There are two main coronary arteries, the right coronary artery and the left main stem. The left main stem divides into the circumflex and left anterior descending arteries. The circumflex artery runs at the base of the heart between the left atrium and the left ventricle. The left anterior descending artery runs the length of the heart at the margin between the left and right ventricle.

Abbreviations: RCA: right coronary artery; LCX: left circumflex artery; LAD: left anterior descending artery; LV: left ventricle; RVOT: right ventricular outflow tract

Myocardial infarction

In contrast to stable angina, myocardial infarction often develops on a relatively small atheromatous plaque which has been insufficient to cause chronic ischaemia and therefore has not developed a protective collateral supply. There is rupture of the unstable fibrous cap over a lipid centre which then induces blood cells to form a clot, sealing the rupture but occluding the lumen in the process.

How is coronary disease excluded?

Imaging

The traditional gold standard is coronary angiography which produces an X-ray image of the interior of the artery with atheroma shown as indentations (Figure 2.2). In uncertain cases, intravascular ultrasound provides extra information about tissue quality over the full thickness of the walls of the artery. Both techniques are limited by showing anatomy and not function. Because of the presence of collateral vessels, it is possible to have a tight anatomical lesion without ischaemia. This is important when we consider the investigation of patients with NCCP to

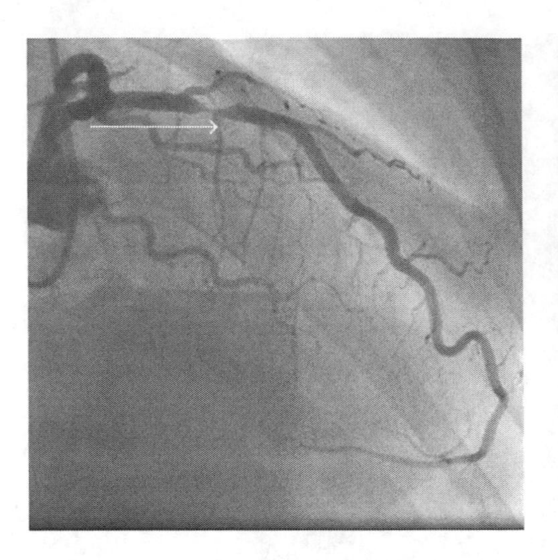

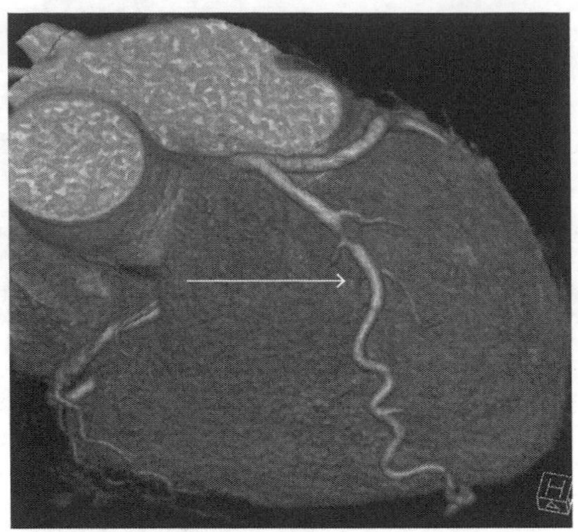

Figure 2.2 Coronary angiogram

There is a tight lesion of the left anterior descending artery (arrowed) shown on invasive dye coronary angiography in 2.2a and on a reconstructed CT in 2.2b.

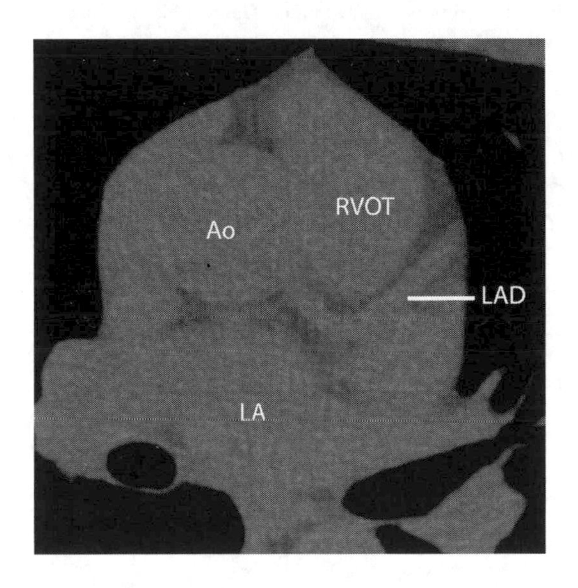

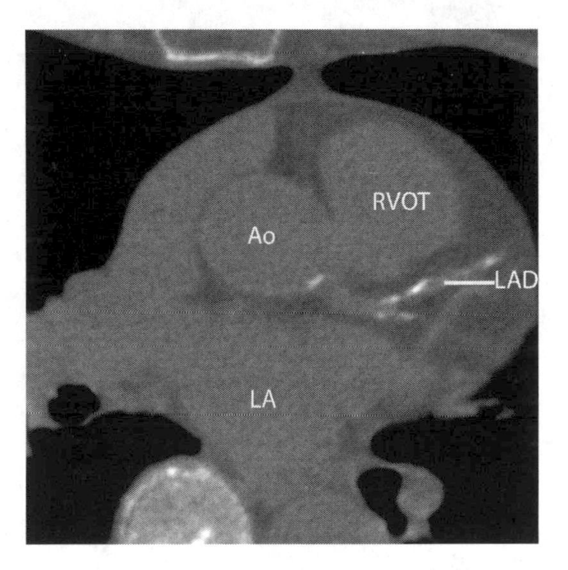

Figure 2.3 Coronary artery calcium

Figure 2.3a shows a normal left anterior descending artery with no calcium, and Figure 2.3b shows an artery with calcium deposits (arrowed).

Source: Images courtesy of Dr Ronak Rajani.

exclude ischaemia. It is easy to misdiagnose the patient using anatomical tests alone.

This is also true of noninvasive anatomical assessment using computerized tomography (CT) (Figures 2.2 and 2.3). CT is a reasonable part of some clinical algorithms but is also frequently used as a screening test mainly at private occupational 'well-person' checks. A CT calcium score gives a guide to the presence of atheroma, and by injecting an iodine-based contrast it is also possible to obtain images of luminal stenosis.

Functional tests

Functional tests are useful since they detect the presence of abnormalities of flow leading to ischaemia, which is the underlying mechanism of angina. The simplest noninvasive functional test is the treadmill or bicycle exercise test, but it is limited in accuracy, especially in women. However, if the patient has non-cardiac sounding pain and good exercise capacity with no abnormal changes on the exercise electrocardiogram, the risk of a cardiac event is very low. Furthermore, it can be used to triage the rapidity with which coronary angiography is needed and can also be used therapeutically as a 'behavioural experiment' or evidence to show a nervous patient that they can exercise without harm. More accurate are the myocardial perfusion study or stress echocardiogram (Figure 2.4).

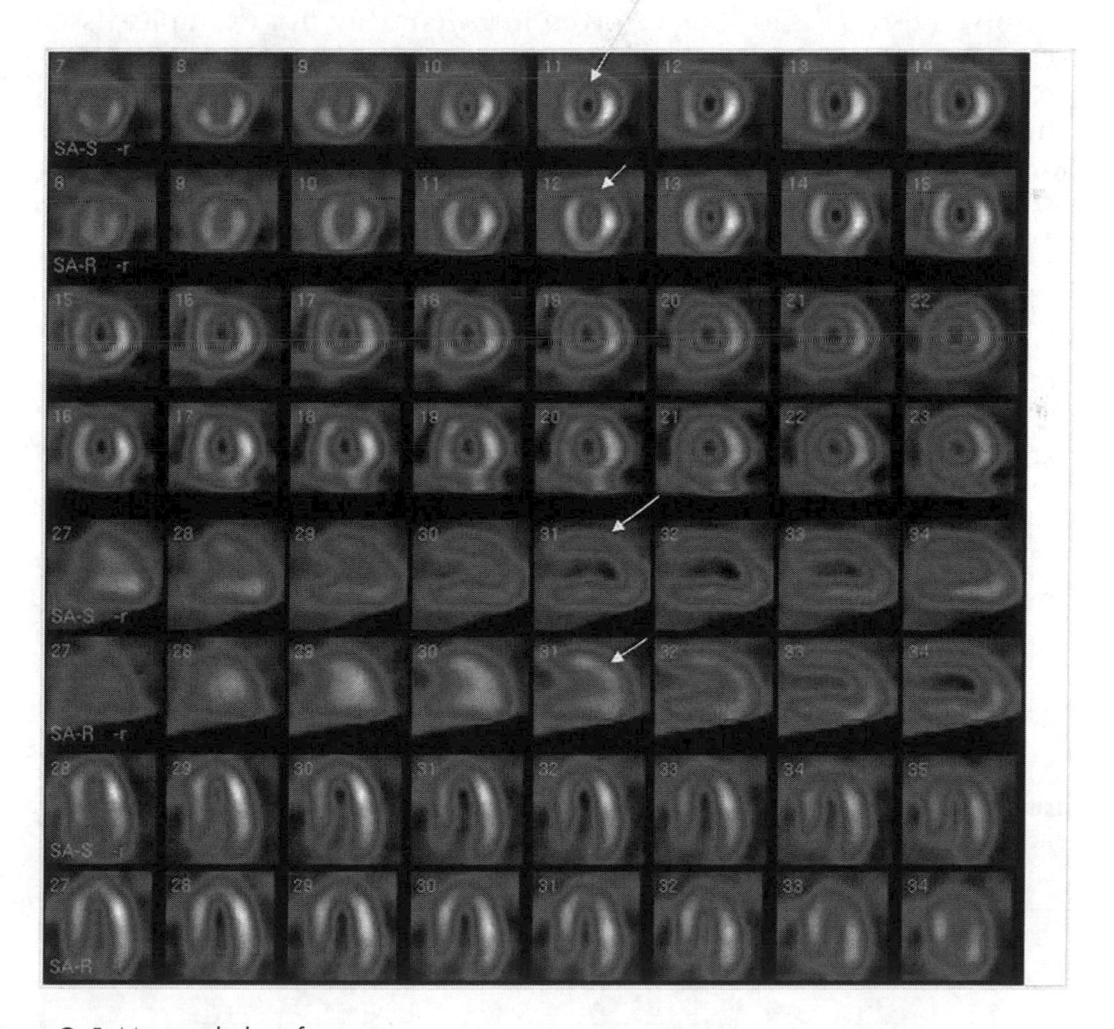

Figure 2.4 Myocardial perfusion scan

There are pairs of sections through the heart at four different levels. At each level, the top line shows the stress images and the bottom line shows the rest images. The top pair is a short axis view near the left ventricular apex, and the next pair a view towards the base of the heart. The third pair shows a vertical long axis and the final pair shows a horizontal long axis. On stress, there is a loss of counts in the anterior wall (arrowed) which returns at rest, indicating reversible ischaemia in the territory of the left anterior descending artery.

Source: Image courtesy of Dr Hosahalli Mohan.

An approach to clinical assessment

The differential diagnosis and the investigative pathways differ according to whether the chest pain is acute or chronic and stable. A patient with acute chest pain usually presents via an emergency department or ambulance. Initial investigation is by an electrocardiogram and a blood test to detect elevated levels of biomarkers (principally troponin, a component of the intracellular contractile mechanism). If the electrocardiogram shows ST segment elevation on the 12-lead electrocardiogram, diagnostic of an acute myocardial infarct, the patient is usually taken immediately to the catheter laboratory for emergency angiography and immediate coronary angioplasty, assuming that an acute blockage or tight coronary lesion is found (Hamm et al., 2011; Steg et al., 2012). If this is not available, then the occluding thrombus is dissolved using a 'clot-buster' given intravenously (for example, tissue plasminogen activator or occasionally streptokinase). If the initial electrocardiogram is normal or non-specific, but the troponin level is high, then coronary angiography is done as an inpatient. If these initial tests are normal, then commonly a noninvasive test like a nuclear scan or stress echocardiography is done, ideally before discharge. Sometimes an angiogram is done anyway as a diagnostic test.

Chronic chest pain is assessed by the chest pain characteristics, the presence of coronary risk factors and the results of noninvasive tests. Chest pain characteristics can be assessed using questionnaires for epidemiological studies (Rose, 1962). However, in initial assessment, the key factor related to the likelihood of myocardial pain, also called 'typical pain', is whether it is reproducibly precipitated by exercise and relieved by rest (discussed in more detail in the preceding chapter). Sometimes the pain is obviously non-cardiac, for example, it occurs in the axilla at rest only. Atypical pain is common and has mixed features with pain precipitated on occasion by exercise but otherwise occurring at rest. The chest pain characteristics and the patients' age and gender can be used to estimate the likelihood of coronary disease (Genders et al., 2011) (Table 2.1).

Table 2.1 Estimated likelihood of coronary disease according to age, gender and character of pain

	Typical angina		Atypical angina		Non-anginal pain	
Age	Men	Women	Men	Women	Men	Women
30–39	59	28	29	10	18	5
40–49	69	37	38	14	25	8
50–59	77	47	49	20	34	12
60–69	84	58	59	28	44	17
70–79	89	68	69	37	54	24
>80	93	76	78	47	65	32

Source: Reproduced from Montalescot et al., 2013 based on Genders et al., 2011

The need for investigation can then be defined according to European Society of Cardiology guidance (Montalescot et al., 2013):

- Risk >85%: coronary disease can be assumed and further investigation is needed for risk stratification rather than diagnosis
- Risk 15–85%: functional test (stress echo or myocardial perfusion scan) or CT
- <15%: no investigation necessary.

In practise, if the pain is not obviously non-cardiac and there are significant coronary risk factors, it is usual to investigate noninvasively. Coronary risk can also be calculated using various web-based systems (for example Q risk: http://qintervention.org/index.php).

Rapid access chest pain clinics

The mortality from new onset angina is 10% at 1 year (Gandhi et al., 1995). RACPCs were established in the UK (Debney and Fox, 2011) to short-circuit the delay between referral from a GP and being seen by a cardiologist. They are usually run by a cardiac nurse under the auspices of a cardiologist, and the target is to see a patient within 2 weeks of referral. At least 75% of referrals to the RACPC have non-cardiac pain, and most have chronic stable pain (Sekhri et al., 2007; Debney and Fox, 2011). In practise, therefore, the RACPC has become the main source of referrals for NCCP to our biopsychosocial programme (Figure 2.5).

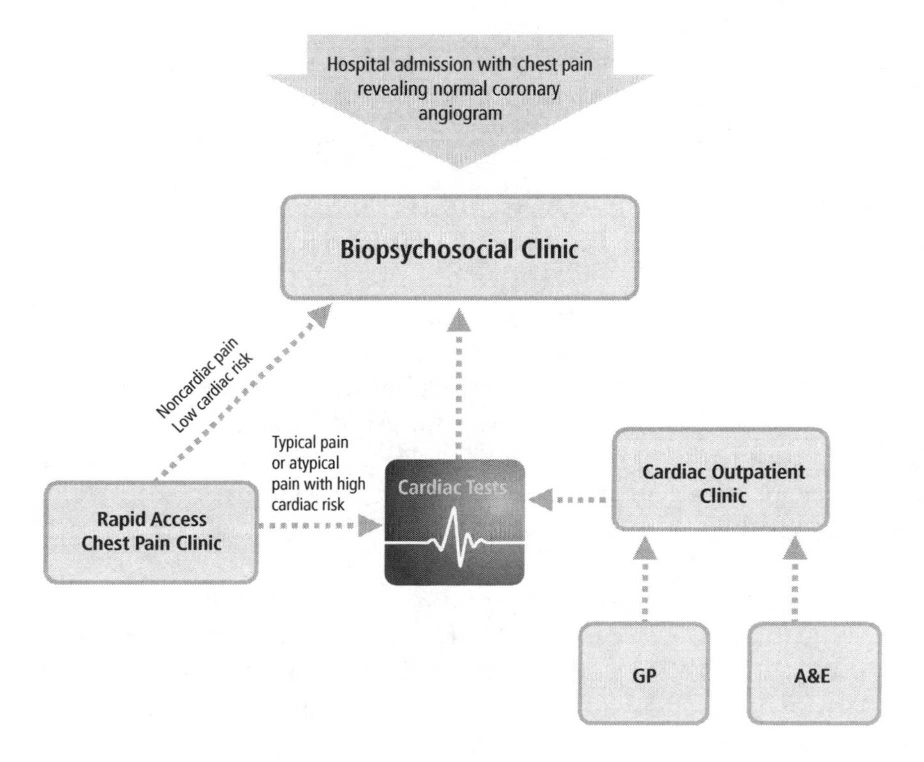

Figure 2.5 Referral patterns to a biopsychosocial clinic

Other alerts that a patient should be taken out of the cardiac management protocol are multiple accident and emergency attendances with troponin-negative chest pain or a normal or near-normal coronary angiogram.

Summary

NCCP can be diagnosed positively if the pain is obviously non-cardiac and the coronary risk profile is low. More usually, our algorithms require the active initial exclusion of coronary disease using a noninvasive functional test, CT scanning or invasive coronary angiography.

References

Debney, M.T., & Fox, K.F. (2011). Rapid access cardiology – A nine year review. *Quart J Med* 105: 2314–7.

Gandhi, M.M., Lampe, F.C., & Wood, D.A. (1995). Incidence, clinical characteristics, and short-term prognosis of angina pectoris. *Br Heart J* 73: 193–8.

Genders, T.S.S., Steyerberg, E.W., Alkadhi, H., Leschka, S., Desbiolles, L., Nieman, K., Galema, T.W., Meijboom, W.B., Mollet, N.R., de Feyter, P.J., & Cademartiri, F. (2011). A clinical prediction rule for the diagnosis of coronary artery disease: Validation, updating, and extension. *Eur Heart J* 32: 1316–30.

Hamm, C.W., Bassand, J.-P., Agewall, S., Bax, J., Boersma, E., Bueno, H., Caso, P., Dudeck, D., Gielen, S., Huber, K., & Ohman, M. (2011). ESC guidelines for the management of acute coronary syndromes in patients presenting without persistent ST-segment elevation. *Eur Heart J* 32: 2999–3054.

Montalescot, G., Sechtem, U., Achenbach, S., Andreotti, F., Arden, C., Budaj, A., Bugiardini, R., Crea, F., Cuisset, T., Di Mario, C., & Ferreira, J.R. (2013). ESC guidelines on the management of stable coronary artery disease. *Eur Heart J* 34: 2949–3003. doi:10.1093/eurheartj/eht296

Rose, G.A. (1962). The diagnosis of ischaemic heart pain and intermittent claudication in field surveys. *Bull Wld Health Org* 2(27): 645–58.

Sekhri, N., Feder, G.S., Junghans, C., Hemingway, H., & Timmis, A.D. (2007). How effective are rapid access chest pain clinics? Prognosis of incident angina and non-cardiac chest pain in 8762 consecutive patients. *Heart* 93: 458–63.

Steg, P.G., James, S.K., Atar, D., Badano, L.P., Lundqvist, C.B., Borger, M.A., Di Mario, C., Dickstein, K., Ducrocq, G., Fernandez-Aviles, F., & Gershlick, A.H. (2012). ESC guidelines for the management of acute myocardial infarction in patients presenting with ST-segment elevation. *Europ Heart J* 33: 2569–619.

Chapter 3

Historical, social and cultural perspectives on NCCP

History of NCCP

Descriptions of NCCP recognizable to a modern physician or psychologist were recorded in 19th century America in civilians and Civil War soldiers (see Box 3.1). Similar descriptions appeared in the First World War (Lewis, 1918; Cohn, 1919). There was depression and concern about heart disease. In Paul Wood's study of 200 military cases (Wood, 1941), the symptoms were breathlessness (93%), palpitation (89%), fatigue (88%), sweats (80%), nervousness (80%), dizziness (78%) and left chest pain (78%). The condition was variously labelled, as da Costa's syndrome (Ogelsby, 1987), circulatory neurasthenia, irritable heart, soldier's heart (McKenzie, 1916) or effort syndrome.

BOX 3.1 SYMPTOMS DESCRIBED IN SOLDIERS OF THE AMERICAN CIVIL WAR (FROM DA COSTA, 1871)

Palpitation

"In some the attacks lasted several hours, and were attended with increased pain in the cardiac region, and under the left shoulder. They were often accompanied by a great deal of distress, and were really painful. They occurred at all times of the day and night . . . The seizures were, of course, most readily excited by exertion . . . But attacks also occurred when the patient was quietly in bed . . . They were variously, sometimes whimsically, described."

Cardiac pain

"It was generally described as occurring in paroxysms, and as sharp and lancinating; a few likened it to a burning sensation, or spoke of it as tearing, or as burning at times, and at others cutting; or as a 'dull sullen pain', becoming at times acute. At times . . . a mere feeling of uneasiness in the region of the heart existed; but in the large majority there was a substratum, as it were, of discomfort, or of dull heavy pain. . . . Deep breathing was stated to make the pain severe, when it was otherwise but slight; cough produced a kindred result."

continued

Respiration

"Shortness of breath or rather oppression on exertion, was constantly complained of, and was a prominent symptom during attacks of palpitation . . . Yet notwithstanding all the signs of dyspnoea, it was astonishing that the respiration was so little hurried."

Nervous disorders

"These manifested themselves chiefly by headache, giddiness, disturbed sleep . . . Dizziness was often complained of. It was increased by stooping; by exercise; and sometimes preceded the attacks of palpitation."

Digestive disorders

" All kinds of indigestions; great abdominal distension, and diarrhoea were symptoms constantly encountered."

The diversity of names arose partly in the absence of a unifying diagnosis and partly because a large number of cardiologists from the UK and the US (and separately in Germany) were recruited to study the condition. It was important as it was the main cardiac cause of discharge from the army. A rehabilitation programme was set up at Mount Vernon in Hampstead, which in 1917 moved to a 700-bed hospital in Colchester. Lewis described their programme of graded recreation and exercise (Lewis, 1918). In addition, "there was plenty of music; in one British camp there were two brass bands, an orchestra, a mandolin, and a banjo club" (Cohn, 1919).

Numerous organic theories of causation were considered including infections, gas poisoning and undetected heart disease. However, a follow-up study in 1925 found that, though only 15% had recovered fully, the death rate was no higher than in the general population, which made underlying cardiac disease unlikely. The condition also became better recognized in civilians, although da Costa had already noted its presence before the American Civil War and many soldiers had symptoms before being called up.

Cohen and White (1951) noted the chronic presence of sighing respiration and a smothering sensation, especially in crowds. Only 24% of Paul Wood's cases could hold their breath for 30 seconds or more. Paul Wood (1956) summarized the consensus that the condition was emotional in origin. In the third edition of his textbook he wrote:

> *It should be understood that there is no essential difference between 'effort syndrome' and 'cardiac neurosis', they are merely clothed differently, the*

> *former in battle dress and latter in nylon. In civil life the condition accounts for 10 to 15 per cent of all cases referred to cardiovascular clinics.*
>
> (p. 237–8)

Cardiac diagnoses often develop over time as a result of new diagnostic procedures. Ultrasound scanning of the heart (echocardiography) is the main method of detecting structural disease. It was first developed in 1953, and unidimensional (M-mode) echocardiography started to be used clinically in the 1960s. It was common to notice an apparent backward motion of the part of the mitral valve during systole, which was labelled 'mitral prolapse'. Patients with possible cardiac symptoms were referred for echocardiography, and many were diagnosed as having mitral prolapse. This led to the concept of a 'mitral prolapse syndrome' (Jeresaty, 1979; Barlow and Pocock, 1984). This incorporated many or all the features previously ascribed to 'circulatory neurasthenia'. However, with the development of 2-D echocardiography, it became obvious that allowing the M-mode beam to scan obliquely across the mitral valve produced an artifactual appearance of prolapse. The realization that the mitral annulus was saddle-shaped meant that buckling of the leaflet in some views was normal and found in a large proportion of normal healthy asymptomatic people (Figure 3.1). Mitral prolapse had previously been overdiagnosed by approximately 20-fold, and the concept of 'mitral prolapse syndrome' faded (Leatham and Brigden, 1980), although it still appears in some lay and even medical texts to this day.

Over-reliance on the results of potentially unreliable diagnostic tests continues to bias the diagnostic process in cardiology as in the rest of medicine. In the 1970s, the term *syndrome X* was introduced for patients with chest pain despite normal coronary anatomy. It was defined by the presence of typical pain, normal epicardial arteries and evidence of ischaemia on any test including the exercise ECG or myocardial perfusion scan (loosely referred to as a *thallium scan*) (Barlow and Pocock,

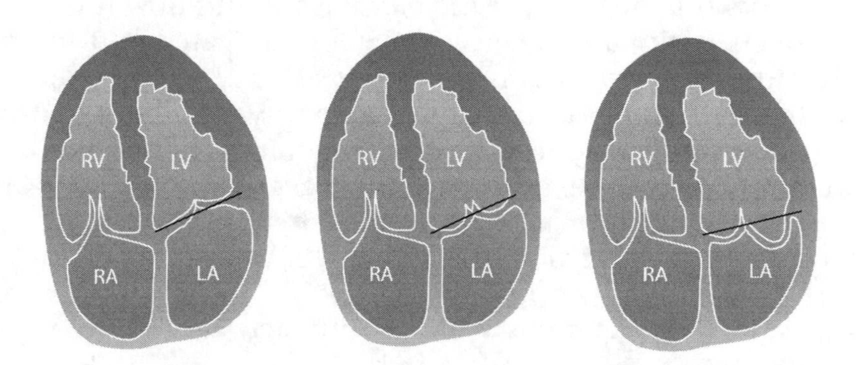

Figure 3.1 Diagrams of the heart to show the mitral valve

The normal mitral valve closes close to the plane of the mitral annulus (left panel) or with mild buckling of the leaflets below this plane (middle panel). This buckling was initially and incorrectly diagnosed as prolapse. True prolapse occurs when one leaflet fails to shut adequately (right panel).

1984). The implication was that the patients were experiencing genuine angina despite the absence of coronary stenoses (see Chapter 2). We have already shown that the definition of typical pain is often imprecise or inaccurate. We now realize that the stress ECG is not a reliable measure of ischaemia, particularly in women, and the specificity of myocardial perfusion scans may be as low as 50%, depending on the technique used. Thus, the diagnosis was made using tests which were not initially realized to be inaccurate. Syndrome X was more common in women, while NCCP is seen approximately equally in both sexes, probably because apparently abnormal ST segment changes are more likely in women. There may be evidence of microvascular dysfunction, but stress echocardiography is normal, and evidence for subendocardial ischaemia on magnetic resonance scanning is contradictory (Kemp et al., 1973; Klimusina et al., 2013). It remains possible that functional stenosis caused by increased arterial tone could cause angina. However, there is an increasing recognition that psychological factors may affect pain perception (Panting et al., 2002; Karamitsos et al., 2012; Parsyan and Pilote, 2012); therefore, psychological treatments should be considered (Rosen, 2001; Karamitsos et al., 2012).

Most patients with normal coronary anatomy have non-cardiac causes of chest pain (see Chapter 5). Thus far, we have considered how there may be a variety of biological factors associated with chest pain and have also recognized the role of psychological factors in the perception and maintenance of NCCP, which is further explored in Chapter 5. First, in order to understand why NCCP has such a profound impact upon people and their lives, we discuss how the meaning of chest pain has been shaped by social and cultural influences.

Social and cultural meanings of chest pain

How people experience chest pain is inevitably influenced by social and cultural factors that affect what the pain means and how it is expressed. Culture affects how pain is perceived, communicated and interpreted. This is because pain perception and expression are moulded by the way that children are brought up within the family, at school and in their broader environments. For example, when an individual has come from a stoical family or culture, they may have developed what appears to be a very high threshold for reporting pain. This can be instilled in early childhood from hearing phrases such as "boys don't cry", or if, after falling, they are told "Get up! You are okay!" As the former example suggests, gender expectations may also impact the experience of and response to pain.

How and whether people communicate their pain to health professionals and others can also be influenced by cultural factors. Pain assessment should include consideration of social and cultural influences; in a clinical setting, however, it is best not to rely on assumptions or generalizations about social, religious or cultural groups, because there is much individual variation within a culture. In this section, we give some examples of the social and cultural meanings of chest or heart pain. When asking individual patients about biological and psychological causes and influences on their pain, it is helpful to find out about what the chest pain means to them and what people in their social, cultural or religious group think about chest pain.

Social and cultural meanings of pain

The word *pain* has a much broader meaning than commonly suggested in medical textbooks. For example, according to the Oxford English Dictionary (2002), the word pain includes the following dimensions, stemming from the Latin term *poena* meaning punishment: (1) an unpleasant feeling caused by injury or disease of the body; (2) mental suffering; (3) (old use) punishment (for example "on pain of death"). In Greek, the word used most often for physical pain derives from roots indicating neglect of love. Another Greek word is *akos*, meaning 'psychic pain', from which we derive the English *ache*. So the early social meanings of pain include the sensations of physical pain related to injury but also meanings implying emotional suffering and possible punishment.

Social and cultural meanings of the heart

Similarly, the heart is imbued with emotional meanings; in fact, the heart is commonly seen as the centre of emotion. The heart image (♥) is used to express the idea of the heart in its metaphorical or symbolic sense as the centre of emotion, including affection and love, typically romantic love. The broken heart, indicating love sickness, came to be depicted as a heart symbol pierced with an arrow (Cupid's dart) or a heart symbol broken in pieces. The red heart image has been used on St. Valentine's Day cards and related products in popular culture as a symbol of romantic love since the 19th century. More recently, the heart image has been used as a verb to mean 'to love', as in I ♥ NY.

We commonly use concepts such as heavy heart (suggesting reluctance), broken heart (loss of love, loneliness), and heartfelt. Someone speaking from the heart is regarded as more credible and having greater emotional authority than someone who merely speaks (Shields, 2002). The heart of the matter suggests the central core role of the heart, and getting something off one's chest implies that problems are centred or held in the chest. The term *heart attack* is commonly used to describe a shock or fearful reaction (e.g. I nearly had a heart attack), again linking the heart and chest symptoms to intense emotion.

Social and cultural meanings of chest pain

If we combine the common social meanings of the heart and of pain, it is not so surprising that chest or heart pain is intensely emotive. When patients with chest pain were asked to freely describe their pain during interviews, they used the following sensory words: "it really hurts", "it is like a pressure", "it tightens", "it grabs", "it crushes", and "it is like a cramp". They also used affective descriptions such as "terrible", "hard and unpleasant", "tiring", "worrying" and "frightening" (Sobralske and Katz, 2005).

Use of sensory metaphors to describe pain has been explored in a study of pain symptoms using an inventory of pain descriptors in six countries (US, Brazil, Japan, China, Finland and Spain) (Crawford et al., 2008). The two most bothersome sensations in the US were burning and electric shocks, while in Brazil they were cramps and pins and needles. The most bothersome sensations for Spanish participants were either electric shocks or "stabbing pins on fire". Interestingly, participants in China defined their worst pain by the emotions they felt or their inability to sleep in addition to the type and duration of the pain episode. In China, the words "heart stabbing", "needle through heart", "tremble", and "bursting" were used to describe chest pain. When speaking about pain, the Chinese participants were more likely to relate extreme pain with the heart because they believe the heart is the most critical and sensitive part of the body (Crawford et al., 2008).

Guillemin (2004) conducted a study to illustrate how drawings can be used to explore the ways in which people understand health problems. Heart disease was reduced to the heart itself, as though the heart was a separate entity, and in many drawings the heart was not even within the body. The majority of the drawings were symmetrical and used the classical love heart of valentines and playing cards. Revealingly, the life-sustaining function of the heart was emphasized: "You can have limbs taken, you can lose a liver, uterus, breasts, bowel, but you can't do without that heart; no second chance". In turn, heart disease was seen as a powerful threat evoking feelings of fear and loss.

The expression and communication of pain can be verbal and nonverbal, both of which have important interpersonal functions. Depending on the type of family and culture a patient comes from, they may have learned to express pain either expressively and openly or stoically and privately. People behave differently with different people depending on the responses of others, such as attention, understanding, ignoring, criticism and so forth. In a study of chest pain experienced in different cultural groups living in the US, Sobralske and Katz (2005) found that members of the Mexican American culture were more likely to use nonverbal pain expression, for example, wincing, groaning and grimacing. In contrast, they found that Arab Americans were openly expressive with pain and that they "may tend to emphasize and exaggerate pain" and "may repeat message for emphasis" (p. 345).

Religion can influence how pain and symptoms are viewed and tolerated. In some cultures, religion is used as an explanation for why people believed they were experiencing pain. For example, Sobralske and Katz (2005) found that Mexican Americans tended to believe that pain is God's doing and God's will, and it can signify punishment. In contrast, for Arab Americans, pain had a more positive meaning as a form of relief; for example, "pain helps cleanse the soul" and "suffering shows courage and faith" (p. 345).

Gender roles and expectations can subtly impact the way that pain is communicated. For example, Menz and Lalouschek (2006) used discourse analysis to examine gender differences in the language used by men and women to describe chest pain. Women tended to focus on the experience of pain and its emotional and relational consequences, while men tended to emphasize its seriousness and focus on trying to delineate causes. The authors argue that such differences in clinical interview settings could suggest gender bias in diagnosis and treatment.

Health messages about chest pain

Chest pain is a common symptom that causes individuals to seek acute care at emergency departments. Since chest pain can be a sign of a heart attack, this association not surprisingly is likely to prompt worry and seeking medical help. As we saw in Figure 1.1, this is present in nationwide health advertising.

An Internet search will consistently produce messages that encourage prompt help-seeking for chest pain. For example, NHS Choices (www.nhs.uk/conditions/chest-pain) says:

> Chest pain can be caused by anything from muscle pain to a heart attack and should never be ignored. . . . You should call 999 for an ambulance immediately if you develop sudden severe chest pain, particularly if the pain feels heavy, pressing or tight . . . . Do not worry if you have doubts. Assume that you are having a heart attack and dial 999 to ask for an ambulance immediately.

Similarly, a US website (www.mayoclinic.org) recommends:

> If you or someone else may be having a heart attack, call 911 or emergency medical assistance. Don't tough out the symptoms of a heart attack for more than five minutes. If you don't have access to emergency medical services, have a neighbor or friend drive you to the nearest hospital. Drive yourself only as a last resort, and realize that driving yourself puts you and others at risk if your condition suddenly worsens. . . . If you have unexplained chest pain lasting more than a few minutes, it is better to seek emergency medical assistance than to try and diagnose the cause yourself.

Prompt help-seeking is obviously important if someone is having a heart attack. However, when chest pain is not due to heart disease, these messages reinforce fear unnecessarily. Visiting an emergency department, with its focus on critical illness, may worsen anxiety. Even if it provides temporary reassurance, fear can easily return. This is more likely to happen if someone has had an experience in which symptoms were diagnosed late or were misdiagnosed and if trust has been eroded. In this case, evidence provided within a diagnostic interview may be doubted, leading to additional opinions being sought. This is why a biopsychosocial formulation and diagnosis is important (see Chapter 7). It also shows how an awareness of social and cultural factors that can influence emotional and behavioural reactions to pain is helpful. A curious, non-judgemental clinical interview can help to explore these issues by gently encouraging the patient to explain their concerns and fears and their experiences and beliefs about help-seeking, as well as their chest pain.

Summary

NCCP is a common condition that affects the majority of patients attending RACPCs. Despite being benign, NCCP has a significant negative impact upon people's quality of life and leads to long-term distress and disability. This occurs even after people have had medical reassurance about their cardiac health. Despite this high level of need, people with NCCP have been neglected by the health-care system, as services focus on assessing and treating cardiac disease rather than offering follow up to people with non-cardiac problems. This perspective on chest pain has developed throughout history and has been shaped by wider cultural ideas about pain, the heart and the potential dangers associated with pain occurring in the chest.

Recent research has explored ways in which health care can begin to meet the needs of people with NCCP, and a biopsychosocial approach is recommended. This requires a broader medical assessment to rule in biological causes of chest pain rather than the standard approach of ruling out cardiac causes. It also requires an understanding of the psychosocial issues that affect people with NCCP and a treatment that can target these issues as well as the medical ones. The next chapter looks at how biopsychosocial approaches have developed and improved our understanding of pain and illness.

References

Barlow, J.B., & Pocock, W.A. (1984). The mitral valve prolapse enigma-two decades later. *Mod Concepts Cardiovasc Dis* 53: 13–17.

Chambers, J., & Bass, C. (1990). Chest pain with normal coronary anatomy: A review of natural history and possible etiologic factors. *Prog Cardiovasc Dis* 33: 161–84.

Cohen, M.E., & White, P.D. (1951). Life situations, emotions, and neurocirculatory asthenia (anxiety neurosis, neurasthenia, effort syndrome). *Psychosom Med* 13: 335–57.

Cohn, A.E. (1919). The cardiac phase of the war neuroses. *Am J Med Sci* 158: 453–70.

Crawford, B., Bouhassira, D., Wong, A., & Dukes, E. (2008). Conceptual adequacy of the neuropathic pain symptom inventory in six countries. *Health Qual Life Outcomes* 6: 62. http://doi.org/10.1186/1477-7525-6-62.

Da Costa, J.M. (1871). On irritable heart: A clinical study of a form of functional cardiac disorder and its consequences. *Am J Med Sci* 61: 17–52.

Guillemin, M. (2004). Understanding illness: Using drawings as a research method. *Qual Health Res* 4: 272.

Jeresaty, R.M. (1979). *Mitral valve prolapse*. New York: Raven Press.

Kemp, H.G., Vokonas, P.S., Cohn, P.F., & Gorlin, R. (1973). The angina syndrome associated with normal coronary arteriograms: Report of a six-year experience. *Am J Med* 54: 735–42.

Karamitsos, T.D., Arnold, J.R., Pegg, T.J., Francis, J.M., Birks, J., Jerosch-Herold, M., Neubauer, S., & Selvanayagam, J.B. (2012). Patients with syndrome X have normal transmural myocardial perfusion and oxygenation: A 3-T cardiovascular magnetic resonance imaging study. *Circ Cardiovasc Imaging* 5: 194–200.

Klimusina, J., Porretta, A.P., Segatto, J.M., Facchinis, M., & Bomio, F. (2013). Cardiac X syndrome: An overview of the literature and the local experience in Southern Switzerland. *Cardiovasc Med* 16: 20–8.

Leatham, A., & Brigden, W. (1980). Mild mitral regurgitation and the mitral prolapse fiasco. *Am Heart J* 99: 659–64.

Lewis, T. (1918). Observations upon prognosis, with special reference to the condition described as the 'irritable heart of soldiers'. *Lancet* 1: 181–3.

McKenzie, J. (1916). The soldier's heart. *Brit Med J* 1: 117–9.

Menz, F., & Lalouschek, J. (2006). 'I just can't tell you how much it hurts': Gender relevant differences in the description of chest pain. In Maurizio Gotti & Françoise Salager-Meyer (Eds.), *Advances in medical discourse analysis: Oral and written contexts* (pp. 133–154). Bern: Peter Lang.

Oglesby, P. (1987). Da Costa's syndrome or neurocirculatory asthenia. *Brit Heart J* 58: 306–15.

Oxford English Dictionary. (2002). *Oxford Dictionaries* (2nd ed.). Oxford, UK: Oxford University Press.

Panting, J.R., Gatehouse, P.D., Yang, G.Z., Grothues, F., Firmin, D.N., Collins, P., & Pennell, D.J. (2002). Abnormal subendocardial perfusion in cardiac syndrome X detected by cardiovascular magnetic resonance imaging. *NEJM* 346: 1948–53.

Parsyan, A., & Pilote, L. (2012). Cardiac syndrome X: Mystery continues. *Can J Cardiol* 28: S30–S36.

Rosen, S.D. (2001). The pathophysiology of cardiac syndrome X – A tale of paradigm shifts. *Cardiovascular Res* 52: 174–7.

Shields, S.A. (2002). *Speaking from the heart: Gender and the social meaning of emotion*. Cambridge, UK: Cambridge University Press.
Sobralske, M., & Katz, J. (2005). Culturally competent care of patients with acute chest pain. *J Am Acad Nurse Pract* 17(9): 342–9.
Wood, P. (1941). Da Costa's syndrome (or effort syndrome). *Br Med J* 1: 767–72, 805–11, 845–51.
Wood, P.H. (1956). *Diseases of the Heart and Circulation* (2nd edition). London: Eyre & Spottiswoode.

Chapter 4

Biopsychosocial approaches to pain

Biopsychosocial understandings of pain and illness have informed our approach to NCCP. Traditionally, pain was seen to conform to a purely biomedical model of disease underpinned by the philosophy of dualism: mind and body functioning as separate entities. The biomedical model meant that diagnosis and treatment would focus exclusively on the organic causes of pain. For cases where the pain was located in the chest, the possibility of heart disease (and therefore mortality) meant that doctors would focus on 'excluding' a cardiac abnormality. This resulted in our current diagnostic terminology implying exclusion: *non-cardiac* chest pain. Such an approach to chest pain is problematic since it fails to recognize that pain involves more than impulses originating in sensory nerves. Other common causes and influences on pain exist and can be successfully modified.

In 1977, George Engel (1977) proposed a radically different approach to medicine based on evidence that psychosocial factors play a critical role in the experience of pain and illness (Loeser, 1982; Waddell, 1987). To understand how psychosocial factors may affect the sensation of pain, it is important to have an overview of the mechanisms involved in acute and chronic pain.

Acute pain

Pain is transmitted by sensory nerves (nociceptive fibres) that carry impulses from every peripheral organ in the body to the central nervous system. This is known as the *ascending nociceptive pathway*. Pain impulses indicate a risk of harm, and when this sensory information reaches the brain, the pain stimulus can be located and a response can be made.

Acute pain is vital to survival because it helps to protect the body from harm. Acute pain arises when there is damage to the body's tissues. Acute pain messages are transmitted by A nerve fibres, which rapidly send the stimulus message to the brain via the spinal column. This is an effective 'alarm system' because it indicates when the body is under threat so the brain can make a rapid response. Responses include changes in behaviour, cognition (thinking and attention) and emotion (e.g. anxiety or fear). Fast psychophysical reactions to the pain alarm are adaptive, as they can minimize harm by ensuring that threats are managed or avoided as effectively as possible. For example, if you cut your hand with a knife, acute pain signals cause you to drop or move quickly away from the blade to prevent further injury. In acute pain, there is an identifiable physical cause (a wound, injury or abnormality) that is medically explainable.

Chronic pain

Chronic pain can be understood as the activation of the body's pain alarm system when there is no acute threat or injury. The term *chronic* is used when pain has continued for more than 3 months (either continuously or intermittently). After this length of time, any physical damage to the body that may have initially caused acute pain will probably have healed. Of course, there are some exceptions, particularly in chronic conditions (such as cancer or arthritis), where pain continues because of nociceptive input to the pain system from ongoing pathological processes.

In cases where chronic pain occurs after healing, the pain messages are transmitted by different nerve fibres (known as C fibres). The C fibres repeatedly send pain messages to different parts of the brain in a slower and more continuous way than A fibres. Such messages are believed to occur when the C fibres develop a pain memory about tissue damage, and they continue to send messages to the brain long after an injury has healed. When it receives these messages, the brain will still interpret them as indicators of current pain. The C fibres are also thought to develop increased sensitivity to other sensory stimuli such as movement, temperature and inflammation. This means that C fibres may begin to send messages which the brain interprets as pain in response to nonpainful stimuli. Together, these changes can be regarded as a *sensitization* of the pain system: an initial phase of acute pain transitions to chronic pain because of changes in the types of sensory messages occurring in the pain system. Messages previously associated with nonpainful stimuli become experienced as pain, which may be (erroneously) interpreted as an indication that physical harm is occurring. Changes in the pain system occur at many levels: in the brain, in the nerve fibres and at the nerve endings. Medical investigations of patients with chronic pain often fail to find satisfactory explanations, meaning that medical treatment is ineffective. As a result, clinicians may conclude that psychological factors are the precipitants of pain, an assumption that is incorrect or insufficient (Jamison and Edwards, 2012).

In chronic pain, since the brain does not clearly differentiate between 'normal' nociception and 'acute pain' stimuli, it may respond as if there is acute pain (and current harm). However, since there is no actual harm occurring, these typical responses will neither resolve nor explain why pain is being experienced, and so the pain persists. The individual will experience this as a failure to reduce pain, and may continue to feel as if the body is experiencing harm. This can understandably lead to negative and worrying thoughts and emotions about the pain. Patients are also more likely to begin to pay more attention to sensations in the body, in an effort to explain their experiences. They may change their behaviour in an attempt to reduce the pain, or they may seek help for it. Unfortunately, these psychosocial changes can further sensitize the pain system.

Biopsychosocial aspects of pain

An understanding of pain that is limited to the biology of ascending nociceptive pathways (including the A and C fibres) cannot adequately explain the complexity and variety of human pain experiences. You may have noticed this yourself with headaches, banged knees, stubbed toes or injections: your degree of pain experienced in these different situations probably varied enormously depending on what else was happening at the time. Psychologists have explored this experimentally by inducing pain in laboratory conditions (using extreme cold or electric shocks), and they have noted that subjective pain experiences differ greatly between individuals. There are reports of far more extreme examples, too, such as soldiers severely wounded during combat who report feeling little or no pain at the time of the injury or immediately afterwards (Best and Neuhauser, 2010).

A large body of evidence has clearly indicated that the pain experienced is not proportional to the degree of tissue damage or physical pain stimulus. Tolerance and sensitivity to pain are affected by many other factors, such as personality (Applegate et al., 2005), gender (Paulson et al., 1998), ethnicity and culture (Campbell et al., 2005), emotional state (Turk and Monarch, 2002), interpretations and beliefs about the pain (Turner et al., 2000) including catastrophizing and fear-avoidance (Vlaeyen and Linton, 2000), and perceived control (Spinhoven et al., 2004). Such factors are thought to influence the efficacy of top-down modulation of pain by the central nervous system (Paine et al., 2009) and the *subjective* experience of nociceptive information through mechanisms such as gate control.

The gate control theory of pain

One attempt to explain individual differences in pain experience is the gate control theory (Melzack and Wall, 1965; 1996). This theory emphasizes the interaction between cognitive, affective and sensory influences in pain. Melzack and Wall suggested that pain messages transmitted up to the brain via A and C fibres must first pass through 'pain gates' in the spinal cord before they reach the brain, and hence one's awareness. Pain gates are said to be controlled by a variety of inputs, including messages from higher-order brain centres and from lower-order parts of the peripheral nervous system. The inputs affect the pain gates (between nerve junctions, in the spinal column and in the brain) and, in this way, lead to heightened or weakened experiences of pain. When the gates are open, pain messages can flow through and pain is experienced; when the gates are closed, the messages cannot pass through and less (or no) pain is experienced.

Messages from the peripheral nervous system, such as nonpainful sensory information coming from other nerve fibres (for example, information about stimuli such as temperature, pressure or touch), can modulate the gates. This explains why rubbing or massaging the site of an injury (for example, if you hit your head or stub your toe) can ease the pain. The gates can also be opened and closed by higher-level information, including psychosocial information (cognitive, emotional, attentional and social learning) (Figure 4.1). For example, pain will probably be modulated by factors such as low mood, stress and anxiety, fatigue, endorphin levels (such as those increased by physical activity) and attentional focus or distraction. Findings that psychosocial factors are a more powerful predictor of outcome in chronic and acute pain than physical or demographic factors (Main et al., 2008) support this theory.

Since the 1970s, there have been many other developments in our understanding of chronic pain. For example, the neuromatrix theory of pain (Melzack, 2005) also posits that pain is multifaceted and involves a complex and widely distributed brain neural network rather than a direct response to nociception and argues for complex changes throughout the body's nerve systems. This theory in particular highlights the significant role played by stress in pain experience. It explains why pain

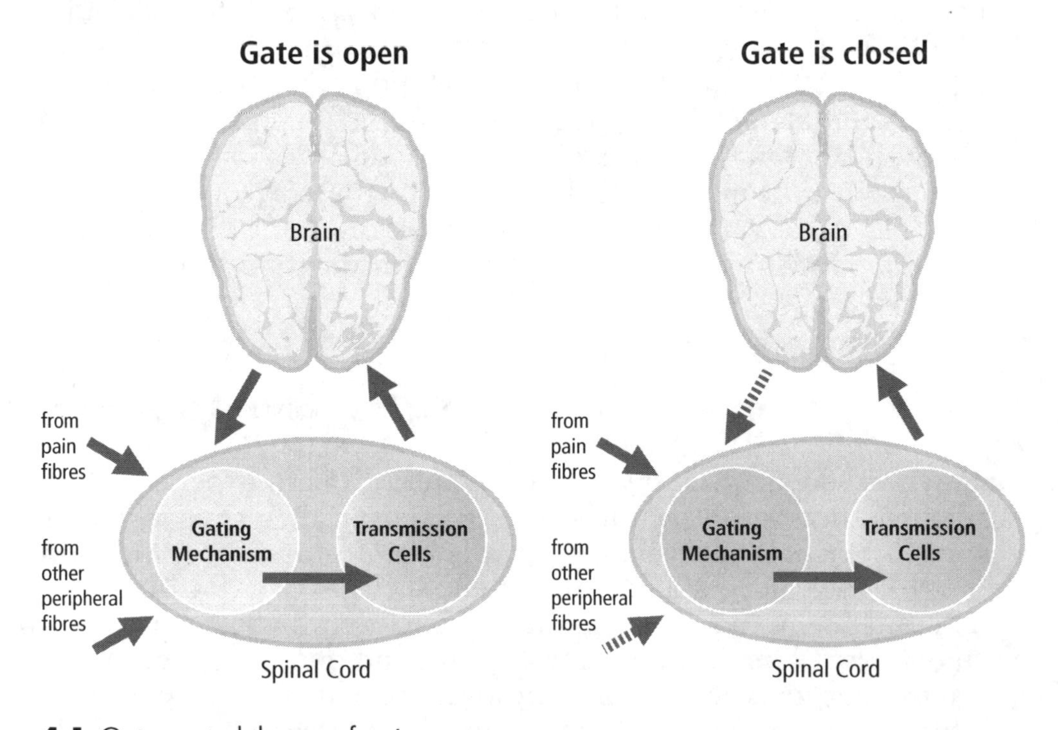

Figure 4.1 Gate control theory of pain

relief is difficult and indicates the importance of developing coping skills for dealing with the correlates of chronic pain. Any coherent model of pain and illness must be able to account for a complex network of interrelationships between biological changes, psychological status and social context (Gatchel et al., 2007), something that a biomedical model alone cannot do.

Cognitive, emotional and behavioural factors in pain and NCCP

Beliefs about pain and current emotional status affect how it is experienced. For example, people with anxiety or depression report more intense pain than those reporting minimal emotional distress (Edwards et al., 2011). On the other hand, people who function well in life generally tend to be better able to cope with, be distracted from or even ignore pain (Jensen and Karoly, 1991). Fear and avoidance are behavioural strategies that can maintain pain in the long term (Vlaeyen and Linton, 2000). These factors have significant implications for our understanding and treatment of patients experiencing chronic pain, including persistent NCCP.

Should an individual hold a strong belief that pain is a sign of illness or a harbinger of death, then treating their pain becomes more challenging. One approach is to learn more about the mechanisms of chronic pain, to moderate beliefs about its meaning and to learn coping strategies. This requires health professionals to offer helpful and correct information and support. Without this, we can see why someone will continue to attribute persistent chest pain to an underlying health threat. They may think the doctors have 'missed something', possibly because they appear to be 'making it up' or the doctor believes it is 'all in the mind'. This misunderstanding between people with chronic pain and health professionals reflects the oversimplification of dualism – that pain is either wholly physical or wholly psychological.

Pain is modulated by how we interpret it, which in turn affects our emotional response and associated degree of suffering. Clearly sociocultural influences must play a role, because the cultural narratives around certain types of pain will affect our interpretations. Chest pain is often associated with the heart, so the perceived threat will be high, sometimes resulting in major changes in behaviour (see Chapter 3). By contrast, pain with a low perceived threat will tend to elicit minimal emotional response, less attention and minimal changes in behaviour. Thus, pain of the same type can elicit different responses depending on how the patient perceives it. Table 4.1 illustrates how different interpretations about the same type of pain might lead to very different experiences of the same nociceptive messages.

Pain involves a feedback process. Our psychological state affects how we feel pain, and our experience of pain in turn affects our psychological state. In chronic pain, particularly if the individual has been given

Table 4.1 How interpretations about pain can affect the experience of pain

Pain	*Thoughts (interpretation of pain)*	*Threat*	*Pain severity and suffering*	*Action*
Headache	I am tired and dehydrated.	Low	Mild	Drink water and go to bed.
Headache	I have a brain tumour.	High	Severe	Worry, can't sleep and go to doctor.
Chest pain	I have heartburn.	Low	Moderate	Drink water and take an antacid.
Chest pain	I am having a heart attack.	High and immediate	Severe	Worry, try to rest, go to accident and emergency (A&E).

a poor understanding of the processes involved, such a feedback loop can continue for a long time. This creates a progressive worsening of the psychological state and the perception of pain. This shows why biopsychosocial approaches to pain (such as cognitive behavioural therapy) are not just effective but are necessary in treating pain (Turk et al., 1983). Evidence for biopsychosocial approaches to chronic pain and NCCP are outlined in Chapter 6.

Summary

Current perspectives on pain do not support a dualistic model of mind and body as separate entities. There is strong evidence that health, illness and pain occur in a social context and develop out of complex interactions between physiological changes and psychological factors including cognition, attention, emotion and behaviour. Key psychological factors in NCCP are discussed further in Chapters 5 and 6. In NCCP, the location of the pain is of particular import because it is commonly thought to be related to heart disease. This offers insight as to why NCCP is often so severe, debilitating and persistent, even in cases where physiological changes are relatively minor and benign.

The next chapter describes the biopsychosocial model with specific reference to NCCP, drawing on experience from our clinic. It is important to remember that in NCCP, multiple processes are interacting, and the different factors involved not only *cause* chest pain but the chest pain itself has *consequences* on the physiological and psychosocial statuses of each individual.

References

Applegate, K.L., Keefe, F.J., Siegler, I.C., Bradley, L.A., McKee, D.C., Cooper, K.S., & Riordan, P. (2005). Does personality at college entry predict number of reported pain conditions at mid-life? A longitudinal study. *J Pain* 6: 92–7.

Best, M., & Neuhauser, D. (2010). Henry K Beecher: Pain, belief and truth at the bedside. The powerful placebo, ethical research and anaesthesia safety. *Qual Saf Health Care* 19: 466–8.

Campbell, C.M., Edwards, R.R., & Fillingim, R.B. (2005). Ethnic differences in responses to multiple experimental pain stimuli. *Pain* 113: 20–6.

Edwards, R.R., Calahan, C., Mensing, G., Smith, M., & Haythornthwaite, J.A. (2011). Pain, catastrophizing, and depression in the rheumatic diseases. *Nat Rev Rheumatol* 7(4): 216–24.

Engel, G.L. (1977, April 8). The need for a new medical model: A challenge for biomedicine. *Science* 196: 129–36.

Gatchel, R.J., Bo Peng, Y., Peters, M.L., Ruchs, P.N., & Turk, D.C. (2007). The biopsychosocial approach to chronic pain: Scientific advances and future directions. *Psychol Bull* 133(4): 581–624.

Jamison, R.N., & Edwards, R.R. (2012). Integrating pain management in clinical practice. *J Clin Psychol Med Settings* 19(1): 49–64.

Jensen, M.P., & Karoly, P. (1991). Motivation and expectancy factor in symptom perception: A laboratory study of the placebo effect. *Psychosom Med* 53: 144–52.

Loeser, J.D. (1982). Concepts of pain. In J. Stanton-Hicks & R. Boaz (Eds.), *Chronic low back pain* (pp. 109–142). New York: Raven Press.

Main, C.J., Sullivan, M.J.L., & Watson, P.J. (2008). *Pain management: Practical applications of the biopsychosocial perspective in clinical and occupational settings* (2nd ed.). Edinburgh: Churchill Livingstone.

Melzack, R. (2005). Evolution of the neuromatrix theory of pain. *Pain Practice* 5: 85–94.

Melzack, R., & Wall, P.D. (1965). Pain mechanisms: A new theory. *Science* 150: 971–9.

Melzack, R., & Wall, P.D. (1996). *The challenge of pain*. New York: Penguin.

Paine, P., Kishor, J., Worthen, S.F., Gregory, L.J., & Aziz, Q. (2009). Exploring relationships for visceral and somatic pain with autonomic control and personality. *Pain* 144: 236–44.

Paulson, P.E., Minoshima, S., Morrow, T.J., & Casey, K.L. (1998). Gender differences in pain perception and patterns of cerebral activation during noxious heat stimulation in humans. *Pain* 76: 223–9.

Spinhoven, P., Ter Kuile, M.N., Kole-Snijders, A.M.J., Hutten Mansfield, M., Den Outen, D.J., & Vlaeyen, J.W.S. (2004). Catastrophizing and internal pain control as mediators of outcome in the multidisciplinary treatment of chronic low back pain. *Eur J Pain* 8: 211–19.

Turk, D.C., Meichenbaum, D., & Genest, M. (1983). *Pain and behavioral medicine: A cognitive-behavioral perspective*. New York, NY: Guilford Press.

Turk, D.C., & Monarch, E.S. (2002). Biopsychosocial perspective on chronic pain. In D.C. Turk & R.J. Gatchel (Ed.), *Psychological approaches to pain management: A practitioner's handbook* (2nd ed., pp. 3–30). New York: Guilford Press.

Turner, J.A., Jensen, M.P., & Romano, J.M. (2000). Do beliefs, coping, and catastrophizing independently predict functioning in patients with chronic pain? *Pain* 85: 115–25.
Vlaeyen, J.W., & Linton, S.J. (2000). Fear-avoidance and its consequences in chronic musculoskeletal pain: A state of the art. *Pain* 85(3): 317–22.
Waddell, G. (1987). A new clinical method for the treatment of low back pain. *Spine* 12: 632–44.

Chapter 5

The biopsychosocial approach to NCCP

Medical perspectives

The first part of this chapter describes the most common non-cardiac, physical causes of chest pain. These include gastro-oesophageal disorders (including neurobiological changes), musculoskeletal problems and respiratory disorders. These problems can often be successfully treated, although it is possible for pain to persist after medical treatment, and we explore this in the second part of the chapter, which focuses on psychosocial influences.

The health professional must be confident that all appropriate tests (see Chapter 2) have been completed to exclude heart disease before they consider using the following biopsychosocial model and the cognitive behavioural approach. The results of these tests will ideally have been explained and discussed with the patient.

Biological (physical) factors in NCCP

Physical factors play an important role in the development and continuance of NCCP. They form part of the vicious cycle of the biopsychosocial model, as shown in Figure 5.1.

Gastro-oesophageal causes of NCCP

Probably one-half of patients with NCCP referred to a gastroenterologist and 5–10% seen in general practise or the emergency room have an oesophageal abnormality as a cause of the NCCP (Chambers and Bass, 1990; Fass and Achem, 2011; Glombiewski et al., 2010; Stallone et al., 2014).

The main oesophageal abnormalities are gastro-oesophageal reflux disease (Figure 5.2) and motility disorders including nutcracker or jackhammer oesophagus (Figure 5.3) (Chambers and Bass, 1990; Fass and Achem, 2011). Nutcracker oesophagus is characterized by high amplitude contractions in the lower oesophagus. A jackhammer oesophagus is an extreme version of this in which the contractions are of very high amplitude, involve the whole oesophagus and have a long duration.

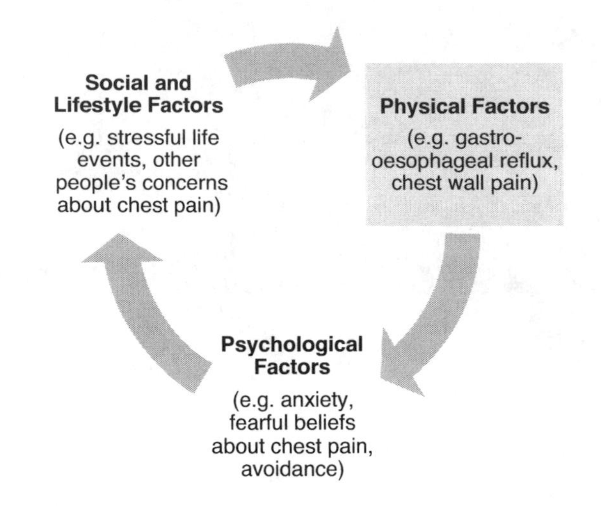

Figure 5.1 The biopsychosocial model: physical factors in NCCP

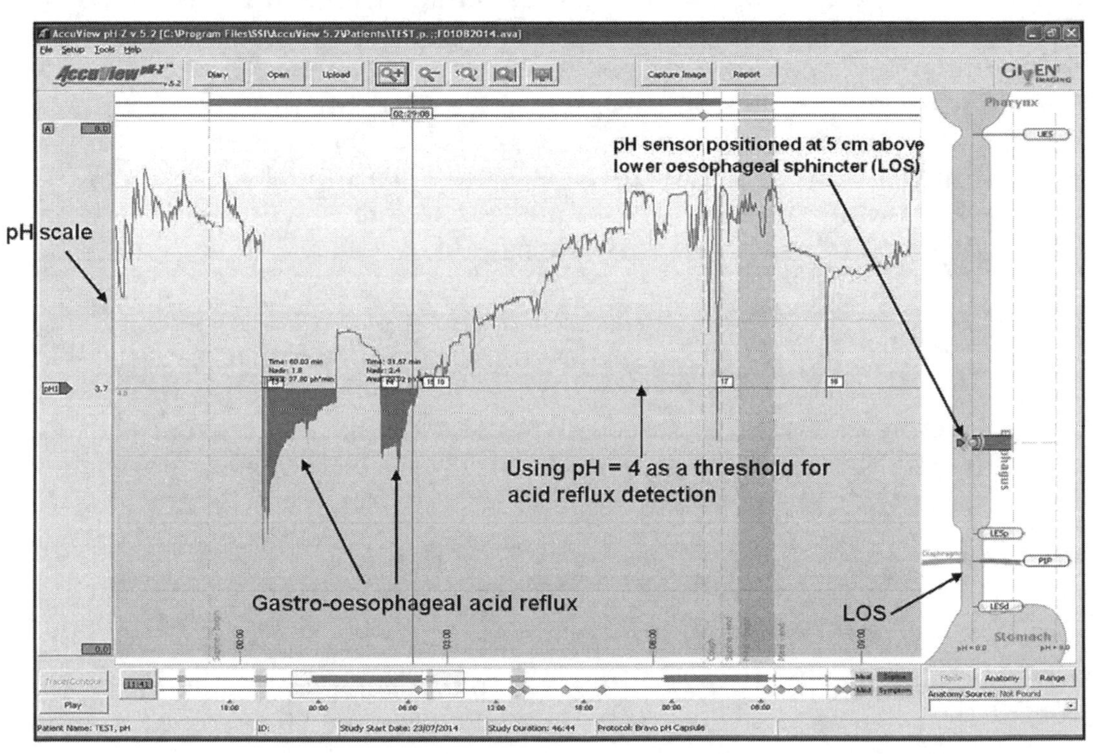

Figure 5.2 Oesophageal pH monitoring

There are two episodes in which the pH drops below 4, indicating acid reflux.

Source: Image courtesy of Dr Angela Angiannsah

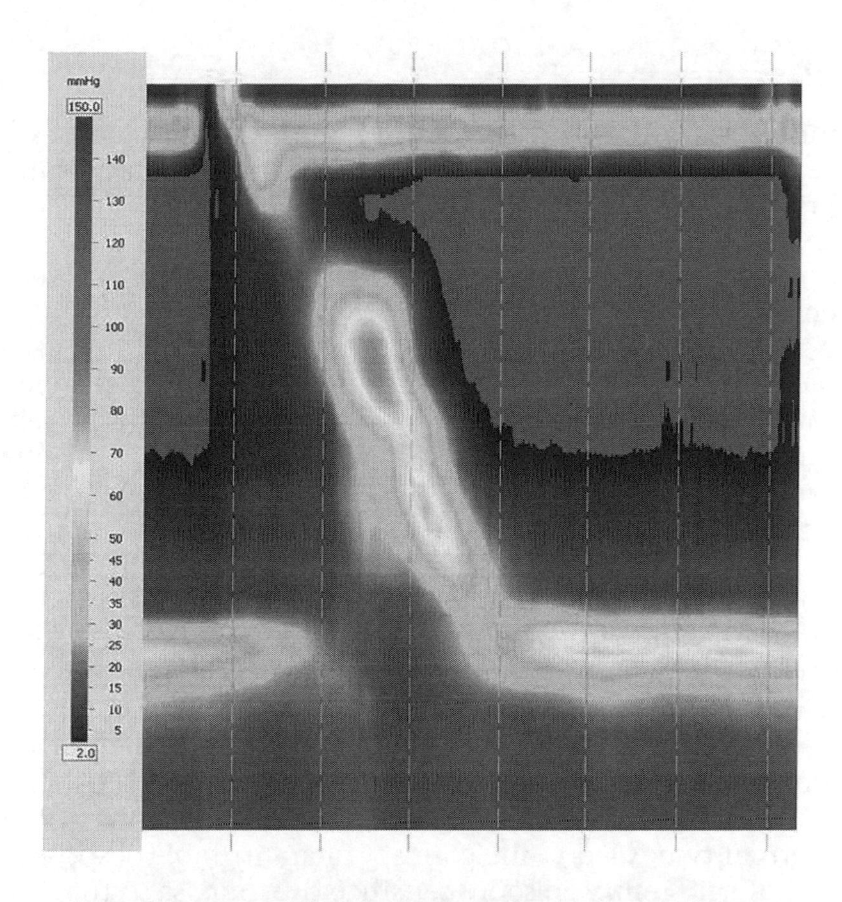

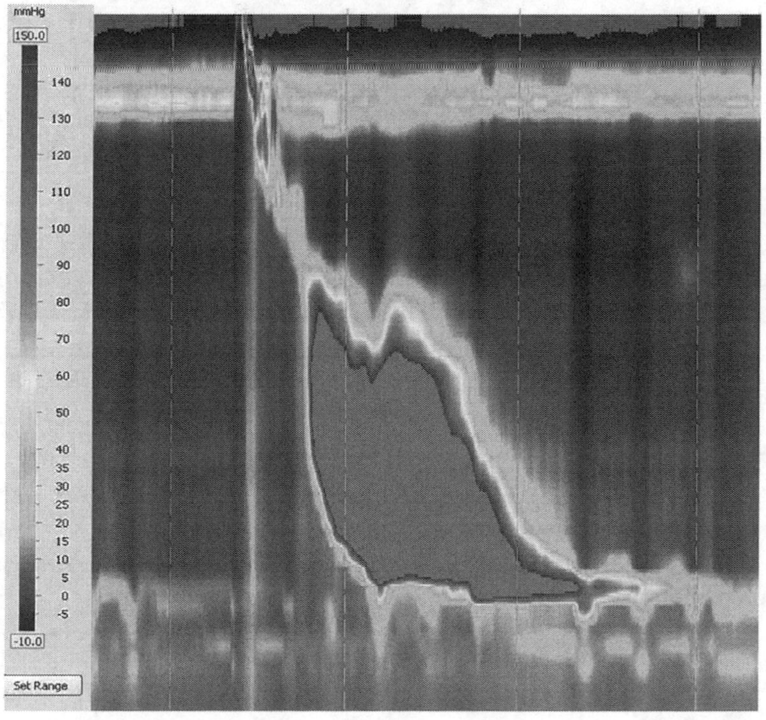

Figure 5.3 Oesophageal manometry

These images show time on the horizontal axis and distance down the oesophagus on the vertical axis. The colours indicate the pressure according to the vertical bar on the left. Figure 5.3a shows a normal progression, and Figure 5.3b shows a patient with hypertensive peristalsis. Nutcracker oesophagus is defined by a coordinated contraction but with an excessive amplitude above 180 mmHg. A jackhammer oesophagus is an extreme version of this in which the contractions are of very high amplitude, involve the whole oesophagus and have a long duration.

Source: Images courtesy of Ismail Miah.

Other motility disorders including the hypertensive gastro-oesophageal sphincter or nonspecific motility disorders defined by a deviation from normal ranges with no clear-cut differentiation from normal. These may be associated with NCCP, but the relationship of episodes of chest pain with an organic abnormality is less clear than with nutcracker or jackhammer oesophagus.

In fact, the relationship between chest pain and an observed organic abnormality may often be loose. Thus, gastro-oesophageal reflux is the most common gastrointestinal abnormality found in patients with NCCP, but these patients may still experience pain with normal levels of acid reflux (Peters et al., 1988; Beedassy, 2000). Patients with NCCP are less likely than patients with heartburn or acid in the mouth to have physical changes in the oesophagus like inflammation or a stricture (Dickman et al., 2007). Similar observations are true for motility disorders. Improving the abnormality of peristalsis with drug therapy may not lead to an improvement in chest pain (Mellow, 1982; Richter et al., 1987). Conversely, treatment with antidepressants has been shown to improve chest pain without correcting the observed oesophageal motility disorder (Clouse et al., 1987).

The poor correlation between chest pain and an observed oesophageal abnormality has led to the concept of an 'irritable oesophagus'. It is possible that acid reflux episodes sensitize the mucosa so that chest pain can then occur with normal levels of reflux. Balloon dilatation in the oesophagus of patients with NCCP causes pain at a lower pressure than in normal people. There is a large literature on abnormal proprioception and central sensitization, which can be induced by many factors including psychological abnormalities (Richter et al., 1986; Mayer and Tillisch, 2011; Farmer et al., 2013).

A mechanistic link between psychological processes and oesophageal abnormalities may be provided by hyperventilation. We induced diffuse spasm or a nonspecific motility disorder in 26% of 46 patients with NCCP and completely normal coronary angiography by voluntary overbreathing at rest (Cooke et al., 1995). Chest pain occurred in 15%, but in none of these did it coincide with an oesophageal motility disorder. The implication is that the motility disorder was an epiphenomenon, with the pain being caused by some other mechanism related to the overbreathing (see next section).

Other abdominal causes of chest pain are rare. Irritable bowel syndrome (IBS) can sometimes cause chest pain by spasm in the transverse colon, and gallstones may occasionally cause chest rather than abdominal pain.

Musculoskeletal causes of NCCP

Between 5% and 30% of NCCP cases (Chambers and Bass, 1990; Spalding et al., 2003) are thought to have a musculoskeletal origin. The wide variation in frequency is caused partly by selection bias, since more people with musculoskeletal pain are referred to a rheumatologist or are cared for exclusively by their GP than are diagnosed by a cardiologist. There is also uncertainty over whether chest wall pain as a result of thoracic respiration or hyperventilation is regarded as a musculoskeletal, respiratory or psychological phenomenon. For example, in a general practice population (Glombiewski et al., 2010) a 'chest wall syndrome' was thought to be the cause of NCCP in 70% of all cases, while a psychological cause was judged to be present in only 14%. Most studies find these frequencies reversed (Chambers and Bass, 1990). However, these distinctions are not terribly meaningful. We have chosen to discuss in the section on respiratory causes since the physiological abnormalities are of the respiratory rate and the end-tidal carbon dioxide content.

Abnormalities of the joints, including cervical spondylosis or arthritis in the dorsal spine, can cause chest pain referred along the path of the somatic nerves originating in the spine (Figure 5.4). Arthritis of the cervical spine is likely to cause radiation down the arms, more commonly bilaterally than in cardiac pain. The pain from arthritis of the shoulder may radiate to the chest as well as down the arm and may be mistaken for cardiac pain, although it occurs at rest or with movement of the shoulder rather than walking. The pain from carpal tunnel syndrome may sometimes radiate up the path of the nerve to the upper arm and occasionally onto the chest.

Chest wall pain may result from bad posture and a careful history may uncover a change in seat or a new computer position. The patient may be carrying a heavy bag across one shoulder leading to a tilting of the spine when walking. Another postulated mechanism of musculoskeletal pain is holding the intercostal and other chest wall muscles taut as a result of anxiety. Chest wall pain may also be a feature of fibromyalgia (Mukerji et al., 1995). This is a diagnosis usually made by a GP or rheumatologist rather than a cardiologist, but the patients appear to share characteristics with many that we see in our NCCP clinics. We await research to see whether similar patients receive a different diagnostic formulation if referred to a cardiologist or rheumatologist.

Chest wall tenderness is often thought to be diagnostic of chest wall pain, although we found that this symptom was reported in similar frequencies in those with normal (31%) as opposed to abnormal (25%) coronary angiograms (Cooke, 1997). However, localized tenderness on examination at rest probably suggests a musculoskeletal rather than a cardiac origin.

Respiratory causes of NCCP

Asthma or chronic obstructive pulmonary disease (COPD) may cause chest tightness on exertion, as well as breathlessness, and this may occasionally be mistaken for cardiac pain. There are usually clues from the presence of wheeze or a productive cough. The cause of chest tightness

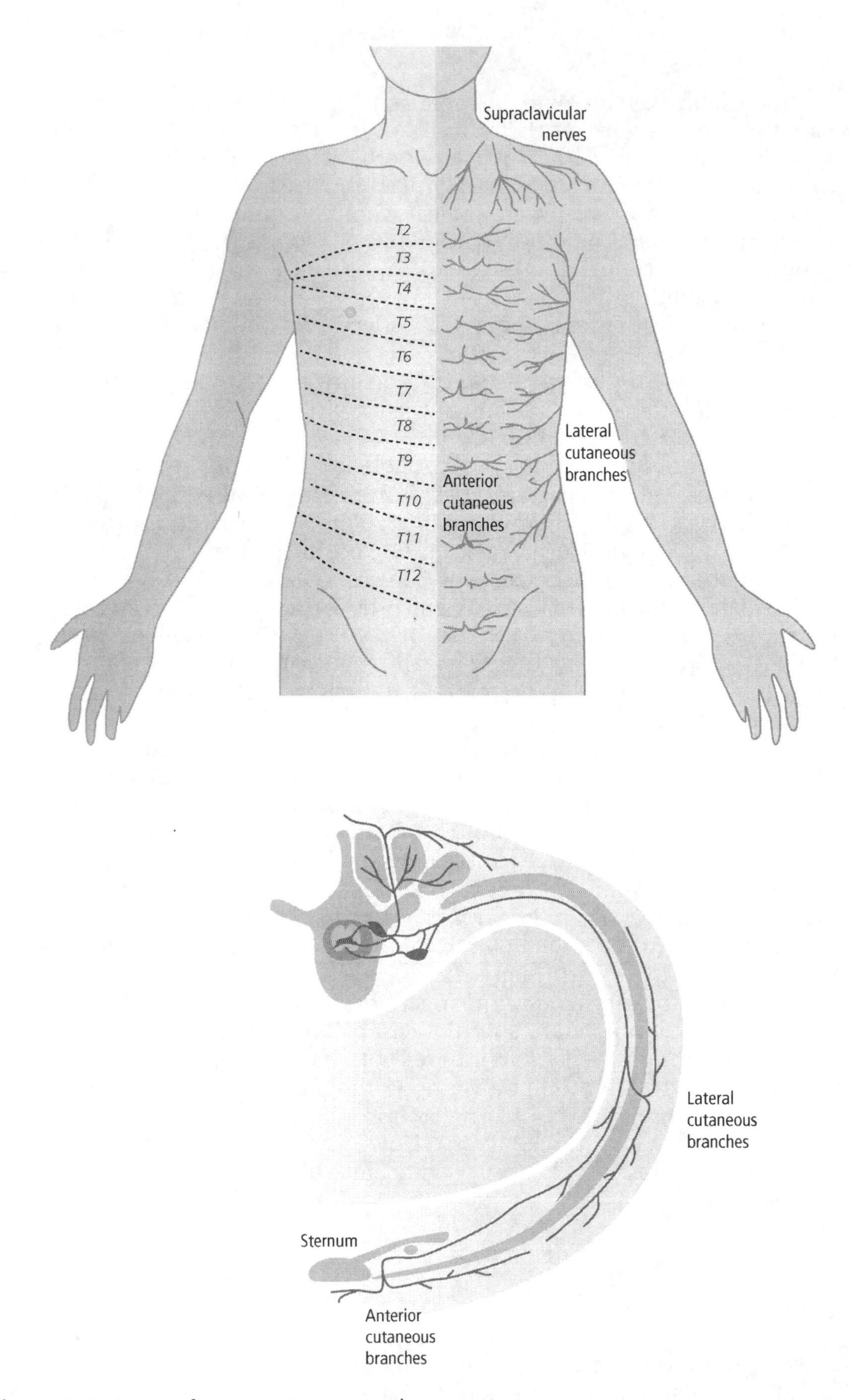

Figure 5.4 Course of nerves originating in the spine

The lower panel illustrates a single nerve originating in the spine and coursing around the thorax. The upper panel shows how these nerves emerge on the skin. Arthritis or other back pathology can therefore cause referred pain in the chest.

in these conditions is not well understood. It may partly be caused by the activation of receptors including rapidly adapting stretch receptors and C-fibre receptors in response to increased airways resistance (Nishino, 2011), but it may also be caused by overuse of the chest wall and accessory musculature in breathing.

Sometimes patients with COPD or asthma breathe with the chest wall muscles even when the airflow resistance has improved, and this can lead to breathlessness disproportionate to the abnormalities on laboratory testing.

A thoracic respiratory pattern can also develop in people without lung conditions. Thoracic breathing is a feature of a panic attack or a normal response to a sudden physical or emotional shock. Recurrent episodes or a chronically persistent thoracic respiratory pattern can therefore occur in anxiety or stress arousal (discussed in the second part of this chapter). Chronic thoracic respiration can also develop after the pain induced by a physical event, including cardiac surgery or a trauma such as a traffic accident. It can result from a change in posture or anything which interferers with normal diaphragmatic respiration, including excess abdominal fat or tight clothing. Often there is a background of chronic persistent thoracic breathing onto which acute episodes are superimposed as a result of an activity or anxiety.

Thoracic respiration may be associated with fast breathing, leading to the movement of larger volumes of air in inspiration and expiration than normal. This is called *hyperventilation*, and it causes a fall in the carbon dioxide concentration in arterial blood and a rise in blood pH. In chronic hyperventilation, the rise in pH is partly offset by increased urinary elimination of bicarbonate, which is alkaline. Low arterial CO_2 causes increased arterial tone with a fall in cerebral blood flow. It also affects oesophageal motility and neural function.

Recurrent episodes of acute thoracic breathing are usually well-recognized as 'hyperventilation attacks'. However, chronic thoracic breathing is less easily recognized. It includes observation of a shallow thoracic respiratory pattern, the presence of sighing and throat-clearing and a short breath-holding time (usually less than 20 secs). The Njimingen questionnaire (Doorn et al., 1982), which consists only of a list of possible symptoms, is insensitive when used on its own. The terms overbreathing, hyperventilation, abnormal breathing pattern or thoracic respiration are used interchangeably. Proof of hypocapnia resulting from hyperventilation is not always sought clinically, although it can be measured easily using a capnograph as part of a respiratory function test.

A thoracic respiratory pattern, sometimes associated with overt hypocapnia (hyperventilation), is commonly associated with NCCP. We showed that air hunger, light-headedness and pins and needles in the fingers, all suggesting hyperventilation, were far more common in patients with normal compared to abnormal coronary angiograms (Cooke, 1997). Such sensations, when arising from coronary disease, may often radiate to the left arm but very rarely to the right. However, in NCCP, it is common to experience right-sided sensations. Most of the patients observed in historical series from the American Civil War and the First World War had a similar symptom complex, and the breath-holding time was short in three-quarters (see Chapter 3). We measured end-tidal partial pressure of carbon dioxide (pCO_2) on treadmill exercise (Chambers et al., 1988). The normal response to exercise is for the carbon dioxide content of expired air to rise during exercise and to fall during recovery, sometimes below normal (4.1 KPa) for a short period during recovery. We found hypocapnia ($pCO_2 < 4.1$ KPa) in 50% of patients with normal electrocardiograms compared to only 14% with ST segment depression and 3% of control people. Failure of the pCO_2 to rise in the first minute of exercise was strongly associated with panic, anxiety and with a history of pain triggered by exercise or by emotion (Figure 5.5). In others with NCCP, it fell below normal during exercise or for longer than in normal subjects in recovery.

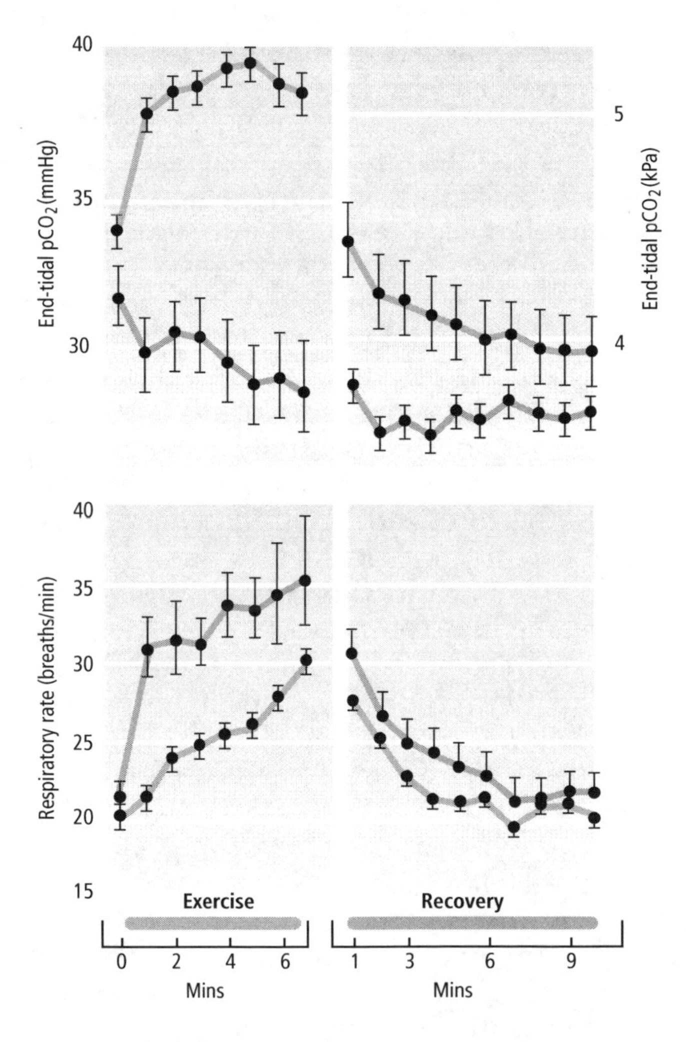

Figure 5.5 Traces showing end-tidal pCO_2 and respiratory rates

This shows the normal pattern and the pattern in patients with initial hyperventilation on exercise. At the start of exercise in the normal subject, the respiratory rate increases slightly but the end-tidal pCO_2 rises. In the subjects with NCCP, the respiratory rate increases more quickly and, as a result, the pCO_2 falls during the first minute of exercise and then further for the whole exercise period. It rises gradually during the recovery period.

Source: Reproduced from Bass, C., Chambers, J.B., Kiff, P., Cooper, D., & Gardner, W.N. (1988). Panic anxiety and hyperventilation in chest pain. *Quart J Med 69*: 949–59.

Thoracic breathing probably causes pain by muscular tension since there can often be associated tenderness consistent in some cases with a diagnosis of fibromyalgia or leading to the suggestion of costochondritis. Costochondritis is inflammation of the cartilage that joins the ribs to the sternum, but the term is often used as a default for NCCP even in the absence of evidence of inflammation. We showed a closer association between pain and the respiratory rate than the carbon dioxide level in the breath consistent with a musculoskeletal origin.

Investigation and treatment of possible organic (physical) causes of NCCP

The patient is often referred for further evaluation of chronic chest pain after the finding of negative cardiac investigation, sometimes following multiple coronary angiography confirming normal anatomy. Ideally, patients should be seen much earlier than this since management starts during the diagnostic approach. Preparing patients for a negative test may make it easier for them to accept simple reassuring feedback from a cardiologist or cardiac nurse. If the chest pain is unequivocally non-cardiac (Guy's Questionnaire score of 0) and the coronary risk is low (for example, using the European Society of Cardiology web-based scoring), there should be no need to investigate, particularly if there is an obvious alternative cause of pain. Treadmill exercise may not then be advocated diagnostically but may still be useful therapeutically to demonstrate the ability to exercise safely. Patients with atypical pain and intermediate or high coronary risk need non-invasive testing, often exercise stress echocardiography, ideally done at the time of the RACPC visit.

Investigation for oesophageal disease may not be useful because of the imperfect correlation between chest pain and demonstrable oesophageal abnormalities. Current guidelines therefore suggest a trial of a proton pump inhibitor for 1–2 weeks to dry up gastric acid (Hershcovici et al., 2012). A referral to a gastroenterologist for consideration of upper gastrointestinal endoscopy or ambulatory pH and pressure monitoring should be considered if:

- There is heartburn for more than 3 weeks.
- There are red flag signs, for example, weight loss, dysphagia (difficulty in swallowing), anaemia.
- Specific treatment is unsuccessful in suspected gastro-oesophageal reflux.

Overbreathing is diagnosed from the history and examination and reproduction of chest pain with breath-holding or voluntary overbreathing at rest. The breath-holding time is measured simply by timing how long the patient can hold their breath in maximal inspiration. This should be longer than 30 seconds, so less than 20 seconds can be taken as unequivocally short. Sometimes breath-holding reproduces the usual pain exactly. We found that 42% of our patients referred from a RACPC had breath-holding times of less than 20 seconds. Voluntary overbreathing at rest is performed by asking the patients to take deeper breathes than normal but at the normal rate. At the end of 60 seconds, ask how the patient feels and whether they have experienced chest pain, breathlessness, dizziness or any other sensation. Sometimes chest tightness is nonspecific, so you need to ask whether the pain produced was the usual pain or a different one. Exercise testing with measurement of end-tidal pCO_2 is a research rather than a clinical technique despite being safe and easy (see previous discussion). Capnography at rest may show abnormally low carbon dioxide levels or an abnormally fast and irregular respiratory rate. The recovery of carbon dioxide levels after voluntary overbreathing may be slower than normal. The treatment of over-breathing is described in session 2 of the workbook.

The presence of wheeze or a productive cough or a family history of asthma or symptoms induced by allergens (e.g. dust, pollen or fur) should prompt respiratory tests including simple spirometry in the clinic. If this is abnormal, the patient should be referred for a specialist thoracic opinion.

Musculoskeletal pain is possible if there is pain or restriction of joint movement. Tests are not usually helpful, although an X-ray may confirm degenerative changes. Treatment of simple uncomplicated arthritis is with analgesics, lifestyle advice or referral to a physiotherapist or osteopath. Patients with more complex problems including severe pain, joint deformities or neurological symptoms should be referred to a rheumatologist. Carpal tunnel syndrome is not a common cause of NCCP, but if this is suspected from pain radiating up the arm, symptoms that are worse in the early morning, sensory changes over a median nerve distribution or reproduced by pressure over the median nerve at the wrist, this should prompt a rheumatological referral.

Summary of medical perspectives on NCCP

Common physical causes of chest pain include gastro-oesophageal, musculoskeletal and respiratory abnormalities. Investigation of the patient reporting chest pain should be extended to include assessment of all of these potential factors when coronary disease has been excluded, or the coronary risk is low or the chest pain is non-cardiac. The chest pain may often respond to specific medication or physical therapy. However, many patients who have experienced NCCP for months or even years may find that their chest pain persists even when the physical cause has been treated. This is because the psychosocial factors affecting chest pain may remain unresolved. For this reason, it is equally important to consider the role played by these other factors in NCCP and how they may interact with the physiological processes.

Psychosocial perspectives

As discussed in Chapter 4, pain is influenced by psychosocial as well as biological factors. Despite this, few clinicians and patients have adopted a biopsychosocial understanding of pain. Pain is often regarded as an abnormality, a sure indication of underlying disease and something that must always be treated and cured. There is very little recognition of the fact that pain, including chest pain, can be normal or a sign of stress rather than underlying heart disease. Chest discomfort is a common experience, reported by as many as 25% in population surveys (Eslick et al., 2002). It is also a common correlate of stress (Chambers et al., 2015; Marks and Hunter, unpublished manuscript; see Box 5.1). In a busy hospital where the pressure is to rule out heart disease, this normalizing stance is rarely taken, and few patients will have chest pain explained to them in this way. Instead, NCCP as a 'diagnosis of exclusion' will be given. Few patients are told what this really means or how they might treat or manage their pain. It is easy to see why many patients remain confused and concerned and why their own view of chest pain remains very focused on biological mechanisms. As with other types of chronic pain, recurrent symptoms are seen as a continuing, even fatal threat from an underlying physical abnormality. This is fostered by the pervasive social and cultural narratives around chest pain that focus on mortality. A vicious cycle of negative thoughts, emotions and behavioural responses (including repeated help-seeking) begins. This maintains and exacerbates the pain. As we saw in Chapter 4, this can affect ascending and descending neural pathways and even lead to sensitization of the pain system.

Researchers and clinicians sometimes refer to persistent chest pain as a type of *medically unexplained symptom* (MUS). Unfortunately, terminology

BOX 5.1 HOW CHEST PAIN CAN BE INDUCED BY STRESS (FROM MARKS AND HUNTER, UNPUBLISHED MANUSCRIPT)

A sample of 625 healthy participants were asked to recall a stressful, everyday situation from the recent past (such as an argument or embarrassing moment) to induce stress and then report on any resulting physical sensations. As one would expect, most people (88%) reported some change in their body. Chest sensations were one of the most commonly reported (by 53%), along with sensations in the stomach (57%), head (56%) and neck/shoulders (52%). Interestingly, these changes occurred in reaction to just thinking about past stress, demonstrating that even the recall of stress can have significant and noticeable physical effects in the absence of external stressors. This can explain why worry and rumination might be have sufficient impact on the body to cause bodily tensions, including chest pain, and they may play a role in the maintenance of NCCP.

This study also provides clear evidence that chest sensations are normal, occurring in a large proportion of healthy people when they feel stress. In NCCP, it is very likely that such normal changes in chest sensations occur in response to stress, and in some cases, this may then interact with other factors to maintain chest pain.

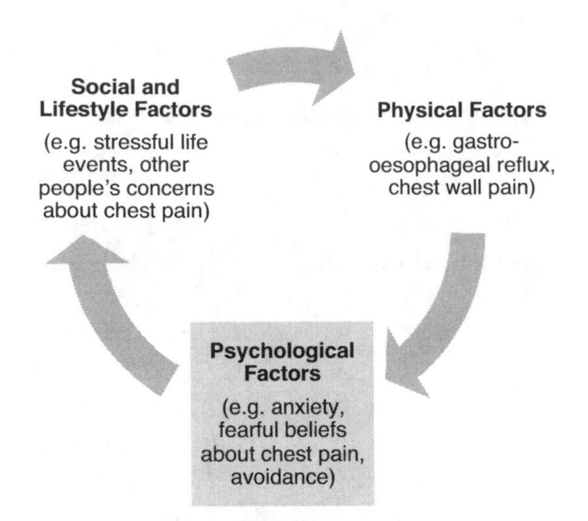

Figure 5.6 Biopsychosocial model: Psychological factors in NCCP. Psychological factors refer to thoughts, emotions and behaviours.

such as MUS is associated with stigma (Marks and Hunter, 2014), since it implies that the symptoms experienced by a person are unexplainable, or possibly even invented. This is misleading and can result in patients and health-care professionals feeling disempowered, as unexplained pain is less likely to be controllable. Researchers have found that terms relating to the idea of MUS often seem incoherent, complicated or ambiguous (Mayou et al., 2005). This is particularly frustrating in NCCP, in which biopsychosocial factors are often explainable and controllable, provided time is taken to uncover them. We would suggest that 'Persistent Physical Symptoms' is a more helpful term (Marks & Hunter, 2014).

In the following sections, we outline the types of psychosocial factors affecting chest pain in more detail. These include cognitive (thoughts and beliefs), attentional (focus and monitoring), emotional (stress, anxiety and low mood) and behavioural (avoidance, safety- and help-seeking behaviours) influences.

Beliefs, interpretations and attributions about chest pain

Chest pain is frequently interpreted as a sign of a heart attack or coronary disease by both the patient and other people (friends, family, work colleagues, even strangers). The first chest pain episode can heighten the sense of alarm if the patient is rushed to hospital in an ambulance. Cardiac tests, even if these turn out to be normal, can be invasive and intimidating. It is easy for the patient to have a vivid memory of a sense of threat.

These intense experiences can lead to unhelpful illness perceptions around chest pain, such as 'I don't understand what is happening to me', 'it is uncontrollable', 'there is really something sinister going on' or 'something terrible is going to happen'. Illness perceptions of causes, consequences and controllability are known to mediate outcomes in

NCCP (and other physical health conditions). For example, when comparing a group of individuals with cardiac-related chest pain to people with NCCP, we found that the NCCP group reported significantly higher scores on panic-type beliefs about having a heart attack. Both groups also reported equal levels of belief in a biomedical model of chest pain. However, the NCCP group reported having a much less coherent understanding of their chest pain (illness coherence) than patients who had a clear diagnosis of cardiac pain. Consequently, those with NCCP found it more difficult to adjust to managing their pain as they were more focused on seeking clarity, and they retained a fear of developing more worrying health problems (Marks et al., 2014).

The persistence of fearful beliefs about chest pain and tendency to attribute chest pains to heart disease has implications for the acceptability of a psychological approach. Patients with NCCP may view psychological approaches as further evidence for the failure of the health-care system to help or that clinicians are suggesting that their pain is 'made up' or 'all in the head'. Cultural tendencies to regard mind and body in dualistic terms neglect the complex interrelationships between health and illness and how physical changes can have profound consequences at all levels of being, not just in the body.

The roles of cognition and illness perceptions are central to the persistence of chest pain. Initial fears about chest pain will not dissipate following negative cardiac test results unless an alternative, coherent and plausible (biopsychosocial) explanation is offered. Unfortunately, the persistence of anxiety can even cause NCCP directly through the physiological mechanisms associated with stress arousal.

Stress, anxiety and chest pain

It is common for healthy people to experience sensations in the chest (pain, discomfort or palpitations) as a reaction to stress. We studied this experimentally by inducing mild stress in a large sample of healthy individuals (see Box 5.1). It may be helpful to share these ideas when working with people with NCCP to demonstrate that chest sensations/pain are not necessarily pathological and are in fact very common.

Stress occurs when an individual perceives a situation as being either outside their ability to cope or as a threat to their well-being. Stress therefore stems from the interaction between a situation and an individual's interpretation of it (Lazarus, 1993). *Stressors* are events that precipitate stress. External stressors may include bereavement, physical or mental illnesses and problems with interpersonal relationships, work, housing, finances and so on. Internal stressors include thoughts, feelings or sensations (such as having high expectations of oneself, low self-esteem or being depressed or in pain).

Stressors only cause stress when the individual perceives a threat (including feeling unable to cope). Susceptibility to stress depends on an individual's genetic make-up, underlying beliefs, sense of self-efficacy,

Table 5.1 Relationship between stress, beliefs and self-efficacy

The table shows how different beliefs about the standards one needs to meet and about one's self-efficacy affect how one thinks about a situation and the resulting levels of stress.

Situation
You have a deadline to complete a report within 2 days. At the same time, there are other ongoing tasks demanded by other aspects of your job that require some attention.

Beliefs about the standards required of you	*Beliefs about your self-efficacy*	*Thoughts about this situation*	*Resulting stress and emotions*
High standards: I have to try to do everything perfectly all of the time.	*Low self-efficacy*: I cannot cope. I cannot do this report perfectly and still do my other tasks.	There is no way I can meet this deadline. I will fail. I will lose my job because I'm not good enough at it.	High stress. High anxiety.
Realistic standards: I want to try my best and make my work as good as it can be within the limits of my abilities.	*High self-efficacy*: I can make a good-enough job of this report, if I set aside time and put my other tasks on hold for a day.	This is a demanding deadline. I will do my best. It won't be perfect but will be good enough.	Low to moderate stress. Minimal anxiety.

knowledge and experience. For example, two people in the same job may both have the same stressors of stringent deadlines and a heavy workload, yet stress is more likely to be experienced by the one with high standards and low self-belief (Table 5.1).

Anxiety is an emotion that occurs when threat is detected, and it is designed to help an individual respond swiftly to that threat. It encompasses a sense of fear, unease or apprehension and anxious thoughts or worries. Anxiety is more likely to arise when we are stressed. For example, if demands at work are so high that you don't feel able to get your job done properly, you may feel stress. Anxiety may then arise if you begin to fear that people are judging you negatively and that you will lose your job. Some people experience excessive, severe and prolonged anxiety that occurs without any obvious stressor, which tends to be associated with mental health problems such as mood or anxiety disorders (generalized anxiety disorder, health anxiety, panic disorder etc.).

When stressors and threats are detected in the environment, there is stimulation of the hypothalamus in the brain. The hypothalamus triggers two neuroendocrine systems that mediate the stress response. One system is the hypothalamic-pituitary-adrenal (HPA) axis. Stress leads to the release of corticotrophin-releasing factor (CRF), which initiates a cascade of physiological changes, resulting in the release of glucocorticoids (such as cortisol) from the adrenal cortex (endocrine glands that lie above the kidneys). Glucocorticoids are hormones that regulate immunological and metabolic functioning in the body. When stress stimulates the HPA axis, the release of CRF leads to many systemic changes in the body. These changes enable the body to cope with prolonged stressors, for example, by increasing the levels of glucose in the blood, to provide fuel so the body can deal with threat. More detailed descriptions of the HPA axis and its role in stress response can be found elsewhere (see Smith and Vale, 2006).

The sympathetic-adrenal-medullary (SAM) system is also designed to respond to immediate threat by preparing the body for rapid defence reactions. The SAM system regulates multiple body systems (cardiovascular, pulmonary, musculoskeletal, hepatic and immune). It is activated from within the autonomic nervous system, which is outside of conscious control. The hypothalamus activates the SAM system so that it releases hormones known as *catecholamines* (adrenaline and noradrenaline). The catecholamines lead to changes throughout the multiple systems regulated by the SAM system and causes the *fight or flight* response. The changes affect the body in a way that helps it to quickly prepare to challenge (fight) or escape from (flight) the perceived threat by increasing physical strength and speed and mobilizing energy resources. These significant changes will be experienced as bodily sensations that we can all relate to feeling anxious and stressed. Note how chest sensations result from a few of these changes (see Box 5.2).

The SAM system activation occurs quickly and stops once the threat recedes. It is seen as an evolutionary adaption that improved survival in environments where danger was immediate and a fight or flight response imperative. An evolutionary example is that of hunter-gatherer ancestors who had to respond quickly to threats in their environment, such as large predators. Anxiety is a fundamental part of being human. It is not dangerous, although it leads to many physical sensations that can feel unpleasant. Without anxiety, our species might not have survived.

In our lives today, we still encounter immediate threats where the most helpful response requires fight or flight (such as jumping out of the way of an oncoming car). However, we also encounter more complex, less immediate threats in modern life (stressors such as interpersonal difficulties, health problems or predicaments at work), which are neither avoided nor resolved by fight or flight. The brain systems responsible for anxiety and threat-response do not differentiate between different types of threat, so the fight or flight response occurs even when stress is chronic, not immediate and not quickly resolved. This can lead to heightened physiological anxiety with associated physical sensations. It can also lead to a reduced capacity to cope with additional stressors.

BOX 5.2 SYMPTOMS OF STRESS AND ANXIETY

To increase the body's capacity for fight or flight, some of the following changes may occur in response to threat or stress:

- Increased heart rate and blood flow to certain muscles so that the muscles have sufficient oxygen and are prepared for action. This results in:
    - Tingling, numbness, coldness and heat in different parts of the body.

continued

- Increased breathing rate to increase the amount of oxygen in the blood, which again is used to power the muscles. This results in:
    - Faster, shallower, chest-based breathing, which can cause chest pain and breathlessness.
- Increased muscular tension as the muscles prepare for action. This results in:
    - Muscle pain, including muscles around the back and chest areas.
    - Shaking or trembling.
    - Pupil dilation and blurred vision.
    - Transient changes in hearing.
- Inhibition of digestion, as the body focuses on using energy rather than making it. This results in:
    - Butterflies,
    - Dry mouth.
- Sweating to help keep the muscles cool so the body does not overheat.
- The need to urinate.
- Increased alertness and looking out for danger. This results in:
    - Increased attentional bias towards negative stimuli.
    - Increase in negative thoughts and catastrophizing.
    - A 'racing mind' and being unable to concentrate on anything else.
- Increase in emotional reactivity resulting in:
    - Fear, anxiety, panic, a belief that something terrible will happen.
    - Aggression.

A diagrammatic representation of this can be found in session 3 of the workbook.

Since heightened stress and anxiety are correlated with physiological changes which include chest sensations and chest pain, we can see how stress alone is sufficient to cause chest pain probably mediated by changes in respiratory pattern, as discussed above. It follows that a reduction in stress could lead to a resolution of NCCP. Usually there is an interaction between stress and other mechanisms of pain, for example:

- Anxiety is associated with fast, shallow, thoracic breathing which can strain the intercostal muscles and exacerbate chest pain. This will be worse if there is coexistent asthma or another respiratory condition.
- Muscular tension that tends to arise with stress can trigger or aggravate pain in the back, shoulders or torso (and this can feel as if it originates in the chest). This will be intensified if there are underlying injuries or other musculoskeletal problems.
- Anxiety can affect the digestive system, for example, inducing oesophageal motility abnormalities.
- Panic attacks are more likely when anxiety levels are high, and panic attacks are often associated with chest pain and fearful cardiac beliefs.
- Stress and anxiety are associated with negative, worrying thoughts, so they may increase vulnerability to negative (and catastrophic) beliefs about the causes and consequences of chest pain.

Attentional focus in chest pain

Anxiety is known to lead to certain changes in attentional processes. There is an automatic tendency to have an attentional bias towards possible sources of threat (hypervigilance). Our culture regards chest pain as potentially dangerous, which encourages a person to notice normal chest sensations while ignoring similar sensations from the legs or other parts of the body. These sensations may then be interpreted as a 'symptom', rather than an incidental normal sensation. Anxiety increases hypervigilance as the person attempts to minimize harm by monitoring themselves and their environment for potentially harmful stimuli. Some patients with NCCP describe how they monitor their chest for unusual sensations and may wear a heart-rate monitor, even when not exercising.

The problem is that, when we look out for a chest (or any other) sensation, we are much more likely to find it. This heightens anxiety and leads to a feedback loop where it seems as if there really is something physically abnormal. Think back to those soldiers we described in Chapter 4 who did not feel pain at the time of their injury on the battlefield; they were not attending to their physical sensations but were focused elsewhere.

You can experiment with the impact of body-focused attention yourself. Spend the next few minutes purposefully focusing on the fingertips in your left hand. Try to notice how many more sensations you can become aware of when you focus attention fully on one part of the body. The mind has limited attentional resources; we can only attend to a few things at once. Sometimes choosing to refocus attention away from pain and onto something more helpful can be a useful coping strategy.

Behavioural responses to chest pain

How we interpret and feel about a situation will influence our reaction or how we behave. Anxiety in response to a threat leads to behaviours designed to minimize the risk posed by this threat. These are sometimes termed *safety (seeking) behaviours,* as they usually involve attempts to avoid or escape potential danger, to seek help or to eliminate the threat. Other interpretations and emotional states can lead to other types of behaviour, for example if we feel depressed, we may be self-critical, withdraw from other people and take less care of ourselves.

If NCCP is interpreted as a threat and the emotional response is anxiety, this will logically result in an attempt to stop, solve or reduce the occurrence of chest pain. This usually means that the individual avoids activities and situations that tend to trigger chest pain, engages in behaviours that ameliorate the pain once triggered or repeatedly seeks help and reassurance. These responses are shaped by cardiac beliefs, and information a person may have gathered about how to 'protect the heart'. As a result, some responses will be based on erroneous beliefs about what will help the pain, rather than because the person has tested out how a certain behaviour actually affects chest pain. The most common behaviours reported by people with NCCP attending our clinic are:

- *Avoiding activity or exercise in general:* This is a common response, based on the assumption that exercise might strain the heart and lead to a heart attack or chest pain. In some cases, activity does trigger chest pain, often related to a thoracic breathing style (particularly if physical deconditioning has occurred from long-term inactivity) or musculoskeletal issues such as injuries that are exacerbated by certain types of activity (such as lifting or moving objects).
- *Resting (sitting or lying down) in response to chest pain:* This behaviour is also common and linked to cardiac beliefs about chest pain and fears about activity. Over time, this can lead to further deconditioning. This response reinforces the fear of chest pain.
- *Drinking water in response to chest pain:* In some cases, particularly if gastro-oesophageal abnormalities are present, people may have found that drinking water can help reduce chest pain, although they may not recognize why this is the case. It can be useful to explore with someone why drinking water might help pain, because this provides evidence for a non-cardiac physical cause.
- *Seeking help from emergency services or GP in response to chest pain:* This is an understandable behaviour when people fear for their lives and remain confused about why their chest pain persists.
- *Withdrawal from everyday activities:* Many patients report significant disability in their daily functioning (for example, stopping or reducing work, socializing less, doing less with their family). This tends to either be because of fear that the activity will damage the heart or because their symptoms are so frequent or severe that they impinge on normal life. Reduced activity is common in depression, too.
- *Keeping busy:* In contrast, some people with NCCP describe how they keep very busy. This may be related to a busy lifestyle or it may be chosen as an intentional coping strategy used to distract from fears about chest pain. In either case, it can lead to increased stress and anxiety.

When these types of behaviours become habitual, they perpetuate chest pain. Reduced levels of activity may lead to physical deconditioning (Rief and Broadbent, 2007) which can in turn increase the risk of exercise-related pain. Inactivity is associated with low mood, depression and stress (Goodwin, 2003). If a patient limits activity because of chest pain, their quality of life, employment, independence and the ability to meet responsibilities will probably fall. This can negatively affect interpersonal relationships, too. The patient may then develop even more negative interpretations about NCCP and how badly it is interfering with life. This adds fuel to the vicious cycle of emotions, body sensations and unhelpful behavioural changes.

Safety behaviours cause additional problems because they stop an individual from gathering information which might disprove their fears. For example, if someone always stops and rests at the first sign of chest pain, they will never find out that they won't have a heart attack if they keep going. Safety behaviours are further discussed in session 4 of the workbook.

Summary of psychological perspectives on NCCP

Common psychological factors in NCCP include stress and anxiety (and the fight or flight response), which have clear physical effects. Psychological factors include cognitive aspects, including negative or fearful beliefs about the causes and consequences of the pain, and an increased attentional focus on the body (especially the chest). Behavioural aspects are important and are usually seen in avoidance or safety-seeking behaviours or distraction. These psychological factors do not occur in a vacuum, however, but will be shaped by wider social and cultural influences.

Social and cultural factors in NCCP

Social and cultural factors also play an important part in the maintenance of NCCP (see Figure 5.7).

Social factors in NCCP include general sociocultural narratives and specific responses in the patient's world. We have discussed cultural perspectives more thoroughly in Chapter 3, where we saw how most cultures understand chest pain to be a profound and worrying symptom that is associated with the heart and connected to danger. In Chapter 4, we also saw how the perception of pain, particularly as something threatening, plays a significant role in how severely pain is experienced.

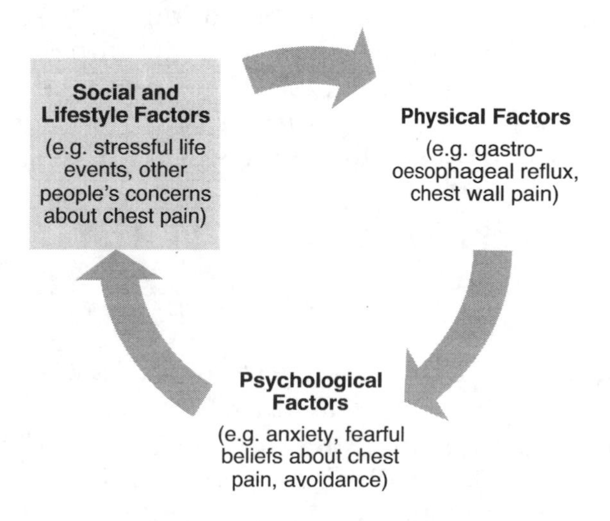

Figure 5.7 The biopsychosocial model: Social factors in NCCP

Messages of risk are repeated in public health campaigns, media and social media. Many patients will describe how family, friends, work colleagues and strangers have reacted to their episodes of chest pain with concern. Initial incidences of chest pain are usually followed by emergency responses (and this may be appropriate). Yet, even after negative cardiac tests, the person with NCCP may find that the behaviour exhibited by people in their social network changes. For example, family members or work colleagues may encourage the person with chest pain to rest or to reduce their responsibilities and activities. This is because *other people* are also subject to social messages, leading them to hold erroneous cardiac beliefs about the dangers of chest pain.

NCCP may give rise to conflict in the social world of the patient, for example, when the impact of chest pain is so great that the patient struggles to meet demands, or when significant people in the patient's life are unable to understand how or why NCCP is continuing to affect them. Lifestyle factors are equally relevant. Life events may cause stress that triggers chest pain, such as bereavement, relational conflict, housing issues, legal problems, financial worries, unemployment or workplace bullying. Other relevant lifestyle factors include behaviours that could make chest pain more likely or make it more difficult for someone to manage psychological distress, such as alcohol or substance misuse, smoking, injury or weight gain.

Summary

Just like other forms of pain, NCCP is a biopsychosocial phenomenon. There are often physical (organic) causes and, just as importantly, there are usually psychosocial processes, too (thoughts, emotions, behaviours and environmental/social factors), and all of these interact. To truly understand, explain and effectively manage NCCP, all such factors must be considered and be understood. With relevant medical explanation and treatment and a psychological formulation of the problem, it will be possible to offer effective interventions that can unpick the components and interactions that maintain NCCP (Chambers et al., 2015). The biopsychosocial approach is explored further in the next chapter, when we discuss cognitive behavioural therapy (CBT) as an evidence-based treatment for NCCP.

References

Beedassy, A., Katz, P.O., Gruber, A., Peghini, P.L., & Castell, D.O. (2000). Prior sensitization on esophageal mucosa by acid reflux predisposes to a reflux-induced chest pain. *J Clin Gastroenterol* 31: 121–4.

Chambers, J., & Bass, C. (1990). Chest pain with normal coronary anatomy: A review of natural history and possible etiologic factors. *Prog Cardiovasc Dis* 33: 161–84.

Chambers, J.B., Kiff, P.S., Gardner, W.N., Jackson, G., & Bass, C. (1988). Value of measuring end-tidal partial pressure of carbon dioxide as an adjunct to treadmill exercise. *Brit Med J* 296: 1281–5.

Chambers, J.B., Marks, E.M., Russell, V., & Hunter, M.S. (2015). A multidisciplinary, biopsychosocial treatment for non-cardiac chest pain. *Int J Clin Pract* 69(9): 922–7.

Clouse, R.E., Lustman, P.J., Eckert, T.C., Ferney, D.M., & Griffith, L.S. (1987). Low-dose trazodone for symptomatic patients with esophageal contraction abnormalities: A double-blind, placebo controlled trial. *Gastroenterology* 92: 1027–36.

Cooke, R.A., Anggiansah, A., Wang, J., Chambers, J.B., & Owen, W. (1995). Hyperventilation and esophageal dysmotility in patients with noncardiac chest pain. *Am J Gastroenterol* 91: 480–4.

Cooke, R.A., Smeeton, N., & Chambers, J.B. (1997). Comparative study of chest pain characteristics in patients with normal and abnormal coronary angiograms. *Heart* 78(2): 142–6.

Dickman, R., Mattek, N., Holub, J., Peters, D., & Fass, R. (2007). Prevalence of upper gastrointestinal tract findings in patients with noncardiac chest pain versus those with gastroesophageal reflux disease (GERD)-related symptoms: Results from a national endoscopic database. *Am J Gastroenterol* 102: 1173–9.

Doorn, P.V., Folgering, H.T.M., & Colla, P. (1982). Control of the end-tidal *PCO2* in the hyperventilation syndrome: Effects of biofeedback and breathing instructions compared. *Bull Eur Physiopathol Respir* 18: 829–36.

Eslick, G.D., Coulshed, D.S., & Talley, N. (2002). Review article: The burden of illness of non-cardiac chest pain. *Aliment Pharmacol Ther* 16: 1217–23.

Farmer, A., & Azia, Q. (2013). Gut pain and visceral hypersensitivity. *Brit J Pain* 7(1): 39–47.

Fass, R., & Achem, S.R. (2011). Noncardiac chest pain: Epidemiology, natural course and pathogenesis. *J Neurgastroenterol Motil* 17: 110–23.

Goodwin, R.D. (2003). Association between physical activity and mental disorders among adults in the United States. *Preventive Medicine* 36(6): 698–703.

Glombiewski, J.A., Rief, W., Bosner, S., Keller, H., Marticn, A., & Donner-Banzhoff, N. (2010). The course of nonspecific chest pain in primary care. Symptom persistence and health care usage. *Arch Intern Med* 170: 251–5.

Hershcovici, T., Achem, S.R., Jha, L.K., & Fass, R. (2012). Systemic review: The treatment of noncardiac chest pain. *Aliment Pharmacol Ther* 35: 5–14.

Lazarus, R.S. (1993). Why we should think of stress as a subset of emotion. *Handbook of stress: Theoretical and clinical aspects* (2nd ed., pp. 21–39). New York, NY: Free Press.

Marks, E.M., Chambers, J.B., Russell, V., & Hunter, M.S. (2014). The rapid access chest pain clinic: Unmet distress and disability. *Q J Med* 107(6): 429–34.

Marks, E.M., & Hunter, M.S. (2014). Medically unexplained symptoms: An acceptable term? *Br J Pain* 9(2): 109–14.

Marks, E.M., & Hunter, M.S. Perception of bodily sensations during stress induction: A survey to inform cognitive behavioural interventions for people with persistent physical symptoms. Unpublished manuscript.

Mayer, E.A., & Tillisch, K. (2011). The brain-gut axis in abdominal pain syndromes. *Ann Rev Med* 62: 381–96.

Mayou, R., Kirmayer, L.J., Simon, G., Kroenke, K., & Sharpe, M. (2005). Somatoform disorders: Time for a new approach in DSM-V. *Am J Psychiatry* 162(5): 847–55.

Mellow, M.H. (1982). Effect of isosorbide and hydralazine in painful primary esophageal motility disorders. *Gastroenterology* 83: 364–70.

Mukerji, B., Mukerjin, V., Alpert, M.A., & Selukar, R. (1995). The prevalence of rheumatological disorders in patients with chest pain and angiographically normal coronary arteries. *Angiology* 46: 425–30.

Nishino, T. (2011). Dyspnoea: Underlying mechanisms and treatment. *Br J Anaes* 106: 463–74.

Peters, L., Maas, L., Petty, D., Dalton, C., Penner, D., Wu, W., Castell, D., & Richter, J. (1988). Spontaneous non-cardiac chest pain: Evaluation by 24-hour ambulatory esophageal motility and pH monitoring. *Gastroenterology* 94: 878–86.

Rief, W., & Broadbent, E. (2007). Explaining medically unexplained symptoms-models and mechanisms. *Clinical Psychology Review* 27(7): 821–41.

Richter, J.E., Barish, C.F., & Castell, D.O. (1986). Abnormal sensory perception in patients with esophageal chest pain. *Gastroenterology* 91: 845–52.

Richter, J.E., Dalton, C.B., Bradley, L.A., & Castell, D.O. (1987). Oral nifedipine in the treatment of non-cardiac chest pain in patients with nutcracker esophagus. *Gastroenterology* 93: 21–8.

Smith, S.M., & Vale, W.W. (2006). The role of the hypothalamic-pituitary-adrenal axis in neuroendocrine responses to stress. *Dialogues in Clinical Neuroscience* 8(4): 383.

Spalding, L., Reay, E., & Kelly, C. (2003). Cause and outcome of atypical chest pain in patients admitted to hospital. *J Roy Soc Med* 96: 122–5.

Stallone, F., Twerenbold, R., Wildi, K., Reichlin, T., Gimenez, M.R., Haaf, P., Fuechslin, N., Hillinger, P., Jaeger, C., Kreutzinger, P., & Puelacher, C. (2014). Prevalence, characteristics and outcome of non-cardiac chest pain and elevated copeptin levels. *Heart* 100:1708–1714. doi 10.1136/heartjnl-2014-305583.

Chapter 6

Cognitive behavioural therapy (CBT) and NCCP

What is cognitive behavioural therapy?

Cognitive behavioural therapy (CBT) is a psychological therapy with proven effectiveness as a treatment for a wide range of physical and mental health conditions. CBT is based on understanding how people think (cognition) and act (behaviour) and how thinking and acting affect emotional and physical well-being. It is a talking therapy, but it involves much more than discussion. CBT is a structured, collaborative effort between therapist and patient working towards clear goals. It utilizes specific skills and techniques that enable people to develop more adaptive ways of thinking and behaving. It is an effective way of helping people understand and manage physical and psychological difficulties.

CBT fits well with the biopsychosocial approach because it deals with interactions between thoughts, emotions, behaviours, physical sensations and the social environment. It is therefore an ideal model for working with NCCP. CBT is not a cure for chest pain, although it can lead to a reduction in chest pain frequency, severity and interference (Kisely et al., 2010; 2012; Chambers et al., 2015b). CBT for NCCP is designed to help people understand why chest pain occurs and persists, to develop more realistic and helpful ways of thinking about it and to learn coping strategies that can reduce levels of distress and disability. Our book is designed to allow the reader to deliver a form of low intensity CBT, also known as *guided self-help*. This adheres to the cognitive behavioural model and CBT principles, which are described next.

Origins of CBT

CBT grew out of psychoanalysis and behaviour therapy and was pioneered by Albert Ellis in the 1950s and Aaron Beck in the 1970s. It is based on the fundamental idea that people are not only affected by external events but also by how they perceive and interpret such events. This is known as the ABC model (Figure 6.1): A (an activating event) leads to B (specific beliefs or interpretations about the event), resulting in C (consequences – emotional, behavioural and physical).

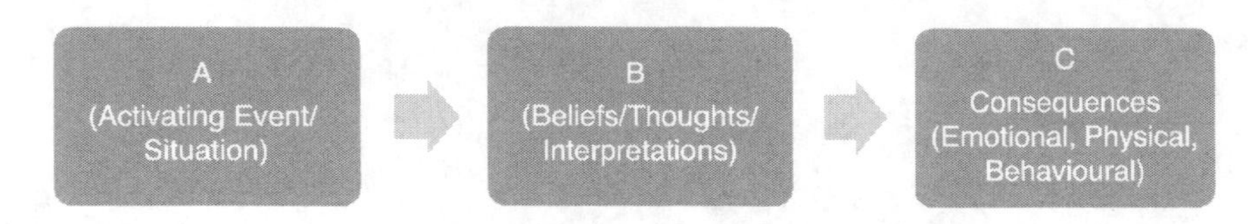

Figure 6.1 The ABC model

Aaron Beck (1979) developed a cognitive model of depression based on the idea that cognition (thinking) plays a central role in psychological distress. He noted how automatic, negative thoughts were common in depressed and anxious patients. This automatic way of thinking would lead to unhelpful emotional and behavioural responses, which appeared to maintain depression and anxiety. His cognitive therapy (CT) approach to depression was designed to reduce distress by identifying and modifying negative automatic thinking. Initial successes, followed by years of research, have proven the efficacy of CT, and it is now a recommended treatment of choice for depression and many other forms of psychological distress. Modern treatments usually involve approaches that change behaviour, too, which has led to the more recent terminology of cognitive *behavioural* therapy.

Cognitive theory and CBT

The ABC model offers a simple explanation of how CBT is relevant to everyone, including patients with NCCP. It can help to use an imaginary scenario with patients to show how thoughts can directly affect emotions and the body, even in an everyday situation. Try it yourself by imagining the following scenario and note the thoughts, emotions and physical sensations arising. Consider what you might do next.

> You are walking down the street, and on the other side of the street you notice somebody you know, a friend or an acquaintance. On seeing this person you wave at them and greet them. This person does not respond. Instead they walk straight past you without acknowledgement. What would you think? How would you feel? What would you do next? Possible reactions are given in Table 6.1.

For many people with physical health conditions, such as NCCP, a psychological therapy, such as CBT, may seem inappropriate or stigmatizing. Using an everyday scenario like the previous one can show that we all see the world differently, and this is why cognitive theory applies to the normal human experience. The way that we think about a situation will affect our emotions, behaviours and even our body sensations. In some cases, particularly if the activating event is particularly challenging or ambiguous, our responses to a situation can become exacerbated and maintained in a vicious cycle (see Figure 6.2 later).

Table 6.1 Three possible responses to the walking down the street scenario

Possible thought (belief)	*Resulting emotion*	*Physical sensation*	*Behavioural response*
They're ignoring me, I must have upset them.	Shame, anxiety, self-disgust	Heart beats faster, tearful	Go home and avoid talking to people.
They look preoccupied; perhaps there is something wrong.	Concern, worry, compassion	Tightness in shoulders	Call them later in the day to check they are okay.
They didn't see me.	Neutral reaction	No changes	Continue with day as planned.

Cognitive theory claims that emotions, body sensations and behavioural reactions stem from an automatic interpretation of a situation. If that automatic interpretation is negative, then the logical outcome is a state of distress. To minimize the distress associated with a situation, the interpretation has to be targeted. This is possible if automatic negative thoughts can be recognized and changed. By identifying automatic thoughts and taking time to re-evaluate them objectively, distress can be reduced. Re-evaluating thoughts requires the person to consider reasons why an automatic interpretation might be mistaken or exaggerated. It can then be replaced with a more realistic, rational and helpful alternative. In the case of NCCP, where the activating event is the occurrence of chest pain, most people report automatic interpretations about there being a problem with the heart, which logically results in fear and distress. An alternative interpretation, based on a biopsychosocial understanding of chest pain (e.g. that this is chest wall muscle pain) is far less negative and threatening. This new, biopsychosocial way of thinking about chest pain should then lead to a decline in fear and distress.

The five-factor CBT model (Padesky and Mooney, 1990) includes all the relevant factors we have already discussed (thoughts/beliefs, emotions, behaviours and physical sensations and social world/environment) in one picture (Figure 6.2). This demonstrates how a CBT model is essentially a biopsychosocial model. As shown in Figure 6.2, each factor interacts with every other factor, leading to the development of a vicious cycle. Thus, a physical symptom such as chest pain, when interpreted negatively (as heart disease), will probably persist, even in the absence of malignant organic disease.

The cognitive behavioural model offers a particularly useful way to explain and understand distress. It is helpful for patients as the factors can be delineated into separate components, which makes them easier to understand and manage. Simple diagrams like those in Figure 6.2 are useful aids for explaining how these components interact and why a single automatic belief (about pain in the chest) can lead to a cascade of multiple changes By reinforcing one another in a feedback cycle, the symptoms persist over time. To see how this applies to NCCP specifically, turn to Figure 7.1 in the next chapter, which shows how a chest pain cycle can be developed.

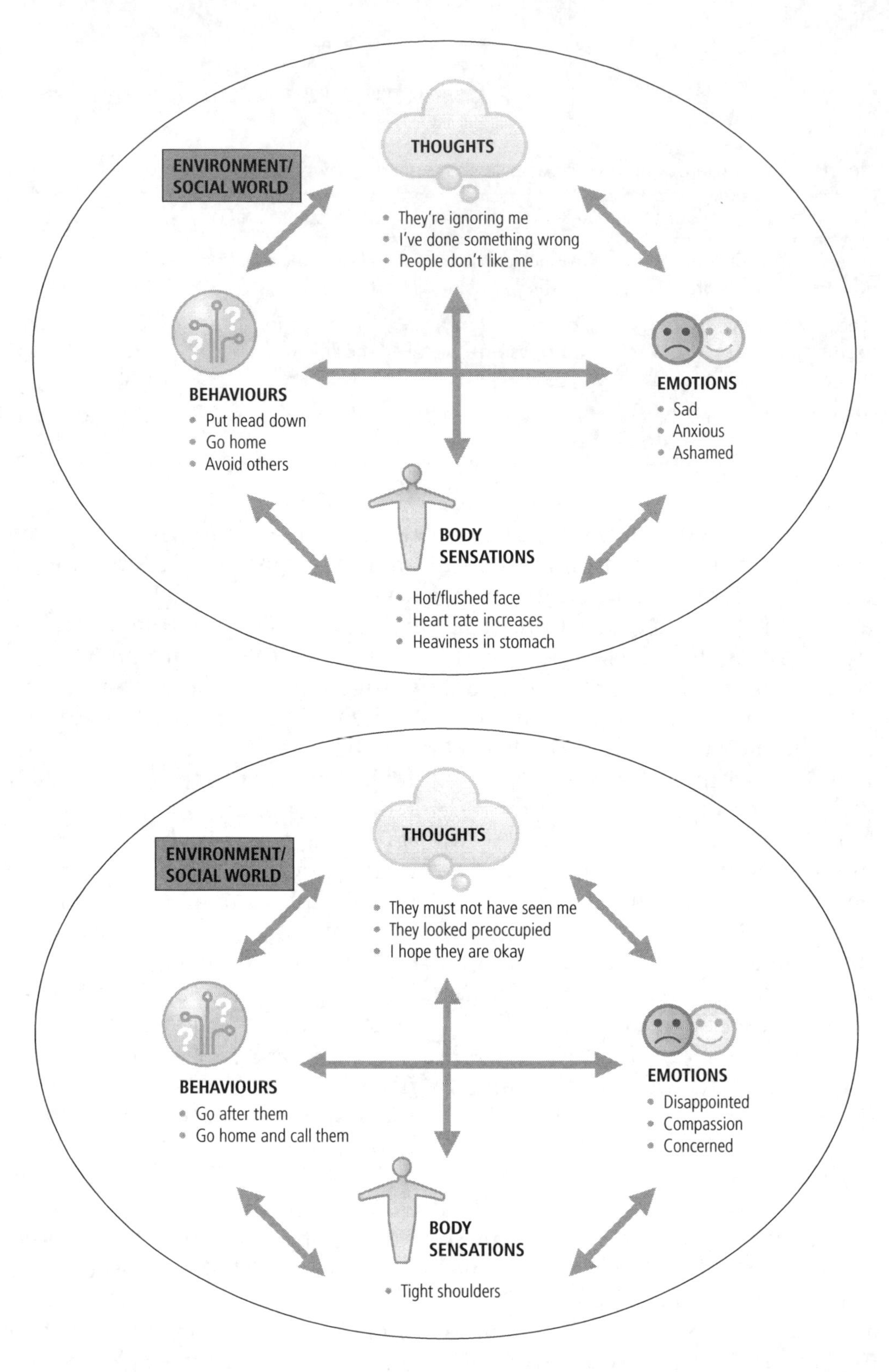

Figure 6.2 The five-factor model

This shows two different possible responses to the walking down the street scenario (based on Padesky and Mooney, 1990). Depending upon how the scenario is automatically interpreted, different emotions, sensations and behaviours can ensue. The interpretation of the situation is influenced by external factors, such as the individual's wider environment and social world.

Thinking styles

Thoughts are not facts. Thoughts often feel factual, but are only ever an *interpretation* of a situation. They are affected by context: mood, past experiences and expectations. Automatic thoughts arise in our minds; they are not deliberate or rational judgements. Automatic thoughts typically happen so fast that we are not even aware of them. Yet we are often convinced by their truth, and we tend to listen to our internal dialogue unquestioningly. We assume that, just because certain thoughts are going through our mind, they must be true. Automatic, intuitive thinking can be extremely helpful. It enables us to navigate the world with less effort, using automatic judgements based on experience and heuristics (rule-of-thumb strategies that reduce decision-making time) (Kahneman, 2011). Unfortunately, this type of thinking can also trip us up and lead to distress because of certain styles and biases in thinking. There are particular cognitive styles where this can be seen clearly, for example, a thinking style focused on threat will characterize anxiety, and one focused on loss and negative evaluations of the self, world and others will characterize depression.

The thinking style can greatly affect the perceived importance of bodily sensations: chest pain in NCCP, hot flashes in menopause or stomach pain in irritable bowel syndrome. Usually, these sensations are interpreted as being normal experiences that are unthreatening, understandable and controllable, so the emotional and behavioural reactions will be neutral and minimal. Yet sometimes people interpret these sensations as symptoms which are anomalous, harmful, unexplained and uncontrollable. This will cause emotional distress (fear, anxiety, sadness) and behavioural changes that attempt to control, understand or avoid the sensations (but which often only make things worse).

Long-term influences on cognition and behaviour

Thoughts and thinking styles vary between individuals. Beck's cognitive model explained how the beliefs people develop about themselves, the world and other people are shaped by their early lives, although they can be modified by later experiences. In CBT, these are called *core beliefs*, and they are believed to underpin the tendency people have to engage in certain styles of thinking and to affect how they interpret certain types of events. For example, someone who has grown up with largely positive messages from family and peers will probably view themselves, the world and other people in a neutral or positive way. On the other hand, someone who has had more negative experiences in their formative years (for example from critical parents, bullying, death and illness in the family) will develop more negative core beliefs. If someone was badly criticized when young, they may believe that they must not be good enough and that other people are cruel. Someone who lost a family member as a child may feel vulnerable in a dangerous world.

Other important factors, including genetic influences, personality and sociocultural context, shape the formation of beliefs. Almost everyone will grow up in an environment that includes a mixture of positive and negative experiences. Indeed, without some early stressful or negative experiences, it may be difficult to develop resilience and coping strategies. People usually develop a mixture of more positive and more negative core beliefs, and their responses to situations will be shaped by the context as well as by their own psychological makeup. Sometimes, negative core beliefs may not play a large role in someone's life until there is a particular trigger, such as a bereavement, relationship breakdown or major illness. In the context of NCCP, beliefs about illness and vulnerability linked to early experiences of family illness may not cause high levels of anxiety until chest pain symptoms develop.

What does CBT involve?

Formulation

The therapist and patient develop a shared understanding of the factors affecting the patient's experience. This is called the *formulation*. Specific thoughts, emotions, behaviours and physical sensations are mapped out from the first meeting, but they will be modified over treatment as further information comes to light.

Therapy

Therapy is guided by the formulation, as it indicates problem areas to target and positive areas to build upon. Goals are set at the start of therapy. Each session is structured by setting an agreed agenda to focus work. Every session ends with a homework task, usually involving the use of strategies or ideas developed from therapy at home. Early homework tasks usually involve monitoring of symptoms and testing out the formulation. Later tasks involve making changes and experimenting with new techniques. Homework is integral to therapy and is reviewed during at the start of every session, providing new information and evidence for the formulation.

Therapeutic stance

CBT is collaborative and the therapist is not an expert but a *guide*, working with people to find out how they can best manage their own thoughts, feelings and behaviours. This fits well with guided self-help.

Therapeutic techniques

CBT is multimodal and might include the following:

- Education/psychoeducation (giving information and evidence about a particular subject relevant to the patient's experience)
- Monitoring and measuring (asking patients to keep diaries and records to find out more about their experiences)
- Behavioural modification and experiments (asking patients to make changes to their behaviour, to predict and record outcomes, and to use new evidence to amend their understanding of their symptoms, attitudes and behaviour)
- Skills training (learning new techniques such as paced breathing, problem solving and relaxation)
- Cognitive restructuring (becoming more aware of unhelpful thoughts and unhelpful styles of thinking and learning how to challenge and change these).

The specific content of CBT depends on the issues at hand. Disorder-specific CBT models and associated treatment protocols are available for mental health problems (e.g. for obsessive compulsive disorder, post-traumatic stress disorder, panic disorder, phobia) and physical health conditions (e.g. chronic pain, chronic fatigue syndrome, tinnitus, insomnia).

Anxiety and depression are commonly comorbid with physical health problems, including NCCP (Marks et al., 2014). CBT for NCCP can lead to improvements in mood and anxiety levels (Chambers et al., 2015a). The application of CBT techniques in healthcare has broad effects on psychological distress.

Common mental and physical health problems treated by CBT

Depression

Depression is characterized by negative thinking styles, negative emotions, low mood and associated physical experiences, such as fatigue. This results in reduced activity and withdrawal from social contact. CBT for depression includes behavioural activation (monitoring of behaviour and mood, and then scheduling a graded increase of activities that engender a sense of pleasure and achievement. Cognitive interventions include learning to identify negative automatic thoughts; gaining perspective by testing out the validity of such thoughts, and then developing more realistic or helpful alternative thoughts and beliefs.

The evidence base for CBT for depression is encouraging. In cases of moderate to severe illness, CBT or CBT combined with antidepressant drugs is recommended (Pampallona et al., 2004). In cases of mild to moderate depression, lower intensity intervention such as self-help and computerized CBT can be sufficient (Andersson and Cuijpers, 2009; Coull and Morris, 2011). CBT has a lower risk of relapse after treatment than antidepressants (Paykel et al., 2005).

Anxiety

Anxiety disorders are characterized by distress associated with anxious thinking (including worry), avoidance, safety behaviours and reassurance seeking. CBT for anxiety focuses on reducing avoidance and safety behaviours. Safety (seeking) behaviours describe types of coping strategies that reduce anxiety when under threat. Effective at reducing anxiety in the short term, safety behaviours are maladaptive in the long-term, maintaining anxiety and fear associated with situations. This is because the safety behaviour prevents an individual from testing out and possibly disproving fears that may be erroneous (Salkovskis, 1991). Treatments for anxiety may also include the learning of anxiety management strategies, such as breathing exercises and relaxation. Cognitive approaches to anxiety are similar to those in depression, and anxious thoughts are identified, tested and modified using discussion, information-giving and experiments using behavioural change. Psychoeducation about anxiety can help to show how anxiety is normal (normalizing), and this often leads to a reduction in misinterpretations about anxiety and its physiological correlates.

CBT for chronic pain

CBT has grown in popularity as a treatment of choice for chronic pain. Although there is no standard protocol, and chronic pain comes in many forms, general CBT techniques include relaxation training, goal-setting and behavioural activation, pacing (learning how to engage in activity regularly without becoming over-exerted) and cognitive restructuring. There have been many systematic reviews and meta-analyses evaluating the efficacy of CBT in pain (e.g. Turner and Roman, 2001; Hoffman et al., 2007; Williams et al., 2012) which all show the efficacy of CBT compared with usual care. Effect sizes range from small to moderate for pain intensity, mood and catastrophizing (negative, catastrophic ways of thinking), increased activity and reduced disability from pain (Ehde et al., 2014).

CBT for NCCP

Regardless of precipitating factors, most patients with persistent NCCP describe changes in cognition, emotion, behaviour and social activity, which are likely to respond to CBT. This does not mean that symptoms are made up, but rather that these very real symptoms are challenging and associated with understandable psychological changes, including negative interpretations about the significance of persistent pain.

A cognitive behavioural, biopsychosocial approach to NCCP can help by first offering people an alternative perspective on their chest pain that reduces fear and anxiety. It can then offer effective coping strategies that reduce the pain and its impact.

Stress is common in people with NCCP, so anxiety management strategies are often needed. Behavioural responses including avoidance often cause significant disability, so behavioural approaches such as scheduling in graded activity are useful. Since levels of distress and disability in NCCP are associated with more negative views about chest pain (Eslick and Talley, 2004), a cognitive approach allowing the patient to develop alternative views about chest pain should lead to improvements in distress. This in turn may result in a reduction in the severity and frequency of chest pain (Chambers et al., 2015a).

Evidence for CBT in NCCP

Various studies have explored how best to help patients manage NCCP. Sometimes it is sufficient to treat NCCP medically. For example, an organic cause such as gastro-oesophageal reflux can be effectively treated using proton-pump inhibitors (Chambers et al., 1998; Tenkorang et al., 2006). Simple behavioural interventions can have significant effects. For example, Petrie et al. (2007) describe how patients who were prepared for a negative result before undergoing a cardiac test were better able to accept the outcome and were more reassured by their cardiologist or cardiac nurse compared to those who were not prepared. Expanded assessment sessions have a therapeutic effect on physical symptoms in general medical outpatients (Price, 2000) and also in NCCP (Mayou et al., 1994) when they include an alternative explanation for pain, unambiguous reassurance and written information.

However, some people with NCCP require more support than just assessment. Meta-analyses conclude that CBT is moderately effective for patients with persistent NCCP (see Kisely et al., 2010; 2012). Standard CBT for NCCP may include education, problem-solving, relaxation, autogenic training (a specific type of relaxation), breathing exercises, graded exposure to activity, behavioural experiments and cognitive restructuring. Evidence exists for individual and group delivery by nurses and psychologists. Most CBT interventions have involved medium-length therapy (ranging from 4 to 12 hourly sessions). Briefer interventions can be effective. Jonsbu et al. (2010) found that a three-session treatment focused on increasing activity improved activity avoidance, depression, fear of bodily sensations and some domains of quality of life, but not chest pain frequency. Esler et al. (2003) found that a 1-hour session of psychoeducation, cognitive restructuring and breathing exercises led to improvements in chest pain frequency, anxiety sensitivity and fear of cardiac symptoms. However, the benefit of a single session was not replicated by Sanders et al. (1997), probably because the intervention occurred too soon after coronary angiography.

Our approach

The rest of this book describes the biopsychosocial CBT-based intervention that we developed for NCCP. It is important to recognize that the book does not train or certify the reader to deliver standard CBT. Offering high-intensity or standard CBT requires extended training and experience. Our book is designed to support the health-care professional to deliver low-intensity CBT, also known as guided self-help, to patients with NCCP. Low-intensity CBT follows similar principles to standard CBT, but it is a simplified treatment. It is manualized and the clinician delivering this treatment should follow a very specific plan, as laid out in the workbook.

Our approach incorporates the best available evidence for extended assessment in NCCP, followed by a brief, low-intensity intervention. As described, a patient's beliefs about NCCP will be significantly coloured by interactions with medical professionals, so treatment begins by offering the patient an individualized account of NCCP that is reassuring and clear. This requires that the biopsychosocial understanding is developed from the outset, so each and every patient meets with a cardiologist *and* a psychologist together for a 1-hour assessment. The individual has a chance to talk about the impact that NCCP has on their lives. This helps the person to feel heard, understood and confident that nothing has been missed. The assessment is followed by biopsychosocial explanations for their chest pain, supported by written information. Medication is prescribed as appropriate.

Stepped care

The needs of patients with NCCP can vary considerably, so our clinic is designed to offer stepped care. In the stepped care model, treatment is offered at different levels of intensity, and patients receive the least intensive level identified by the clinician as being likely to benefit them. Patients can be stepped up if further support is found to be necessary (see Bower and Gilbody, 2005, for a review). Figure 6.3 demonstrates how a stepped care intervention can be designed.

Following assessment (and sometimes medication), there are three possible steps of care. This is possible because we have both a clinical psychologist and cardiac nurses.

- Step 1: No further intervention, with a follow-up telephone call at 2 weeks.
- Step 2: Guided self-help (low intensity CBT); up to 5 sessions of guided self-help with a cardiac nurse.
- Step 3: High intensity CBT; up to 8 sessions of standard CBT with a clinical psychologist (or CBT therapist).

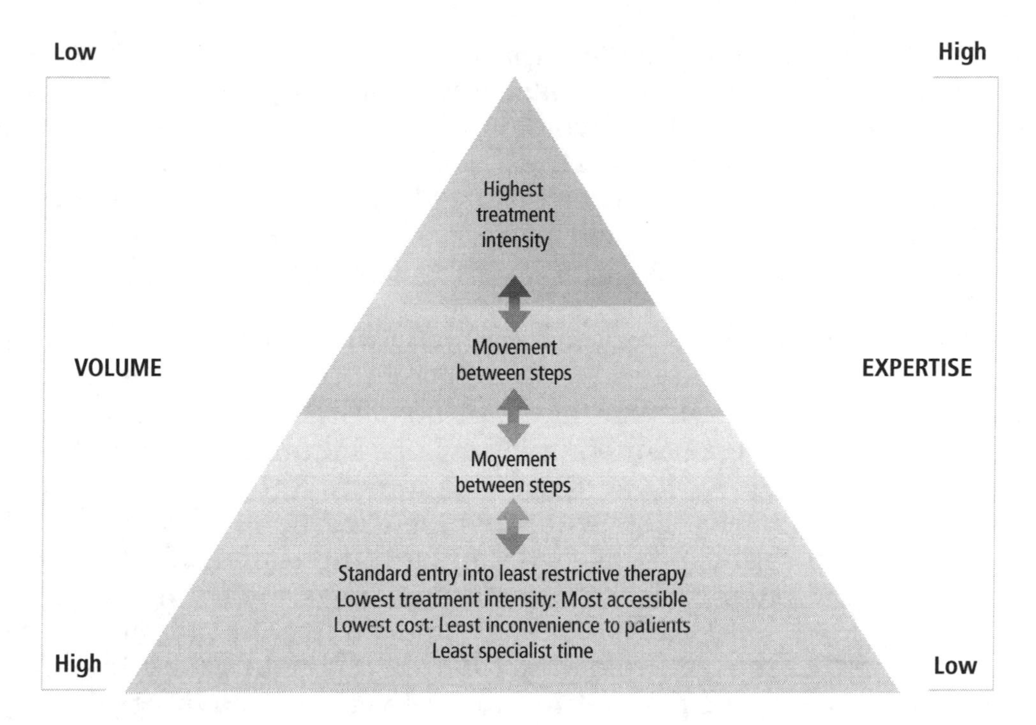

Figure 6.3 Stepped care

Source: Adapted from Espie (2009) and reproduced with kind permission from the American Academy of Sleep Medicine.

The step offered is based on our clinical judgement of the severity of the problem. Patients reporting mild to moderate distress are offered guided self-help with a cardiac nurse. Patients reporting more severe distress and/or complex comorbidities are offered high intensity CBT with a clinical psychologist. It is possible for patients to move between steps. For example, if more complex issues arise during guided self-help, the patient can be moved to step 3. If patients respond swiftly to high-intensity CBT, the psychologist may step down to guided self-help (described in the workbook section).

Outcomes from our clinic

Over a 1-year period, we assessed and treated 77 people with a diagnosis of NCCP. Most were referred from a RACPC, and all had been experiencing NCCP that occurred at least once a month (usually much more frequently) for at least 3 months and were significantly distressed. Our treatment was acceptable and effective, with low drop-out rates (Chambers et al., 2015a; Marks et al., 2016). We found beneficial changes in a number of areas, from baseline to the end of treatment, which were maintained at the 6-month follow up:

- Chest pain frequency of at least once a month was reported by 100% of patients at baseline. This reduced to 51% of patients at 6-month follow up.

- Chest pain interference significantly reduced.
- Negative (cardiac) beliefs significantly reduced.
- The percentage of patients avoiding activity reduced (from 66% to 9%).
- Anxiety reduced (from 42% to 16% of people meeting 'caseness').
- Depression reduced (from 34% to 15% of people meeting 'caseness').
- Improvements in functioning were reported, with reductions in work absenteeism and lower use of health-care resources.

Our outcomes compare very favourably with those from other studies using more intensive CBT, which have reported reductions in chest pain frequency in the range of 50–69%. Due to our stepped-care model, the average number of sessions required by patients was just three, which is far lower than the standard 8–12 sessions of high intensity CBT described elsewhere. Guided self-help (step 2) was sufficient for 43%, while 44% needed standard (high-intensity) CBT with a psychologist (step 3), and 13% required assessment only (step 1). Clearly, guided self-help has broad applicability and is relevant in today's health services. Guided self-help is a low-intensity intervention and hence can be manualized and delivered effectively by a range of health care professionals who may not have full training in CBT, although they will need to access CBT supervision.

The study described here was a clinical evaluation and not a randomized controlled trial. Yet the results still suggest that our treatment is likely to be more effective than treatment as usual. In the UK, where usual treatment for NCCP involves testing to exclude cardiac disease followed by GP care, treatment as usual tends to result in long-term distress, disability and persistent chest pain (Marks et al., 2014). Biopsychosocial assessment followed by a CBT-informed intervention, however, offers a chance to change this, providing people with a new way to improve and manage NCCP and possibly even recover from it. We hope that our book can help to make this brief CBT-based treatment more accessible to people with NCCP and their health-care providers.

The next chapter teaches the reader to conduct biopsychosocial assessment of chest pain and discusses how to formulate this in a CBT model. In the second section of the book, we offer the reader a step-by-step treatment workbook to follow with patients in the form of guided self-help.

References

Andersson, G., & Cuijpers, P. (2009). Internet-based and other computerized psychological treatments for adult depression: A meta-analysis. *Cogn Behav Ther* 38(4): 196–205.

Beck, A.T. ed. (1979). *Cognitive therapy of depression*. New York, NY: Guilford Press.

Bower, P., & Gilbody, S. (2005). Stepped care in psychological therapies: Access, effectiveness and efficiency. *Br J Psychiatry* 186(1): 11–17.

Chambers, J.B., Cooke, R., Anggiansah, A., & Owen, W. (1998). Effects of omeprazole in patients with chest pain and normal coronary anatomy: Initial experience. *Int J Cardiol* 65: 51–5.

Chambers, J.B., Marks, E.M., & Hunter, M.S. (2015a). The head says yes but the heart says no: What is non-cardiac chest pain and how is it managed? *Heart Educ* 101: 1240–9.

Chambers, J.B., Marks, E.M., Russell, V., & Hunter, M.S. (2015b). A multidisciplinary, biopsychosocial treatment for non-cardiac chest pain. *Int J Cardiol* 69(9): 922–7.

Clark, D.M., Layard, R., Smithies, R., Richards, D.A., Suckling, R., & Wright, B. (2009). Improving access to psychological therapy: Initial evaluation of two UK demonstration sites. *Behav Res Ther* 47(11): 910–20.

Coull, G., & Morris, P.G. (2011). The clinical effectiveness of CBT-based guided self-help interventions for anxiety and depressive disorders: A systematic review. *Psychol Med* 41(11): 2239.

Ehde, D.M., Dillworth, T.M., & Turner, J.A. (2014). Cognitive-behavioral therapy for individuals with chronic pain: Efficacy, innovations, and directions for research. *Am Psychol* 69(2): 153.

Esler, J.L., Barlow, D.H., Woolard, R.H., Nicholson, R.A., Nash, J.M., & Erogul, M.H. (2003). A brief cognitive-behavioral intervention for patients with noncardiac chest pain. *Behav Ther* 34: 129–48.

Eslick, G.D., & Talley, N.J. (2004). Non-cardiac chest pain: Predictors of health care seeking, the types of health care professional consulted, work absenteeism and interruption of daily activities. *Aliment Pharmacol Ther* 20: 909–15.

Espie, C.A. (2009). 'Stepped care': A health technology solution for delivering cognitive behavioral therapy as a first line insomnia treatment. *SLEEP* 32(12): 1549–58.

Hoffman, B.M., Papas, R.K., Chatkoff, D.K., & Kerns, R.D. (2007). Meta-analysis of psychological interventions for chronic low back pain. *Health Psychol* 26(1): 1–9.

Jonsbu, E., Dammen, T., Morken, G., Moum, T., & Martinsen, E.W. (2010). Short term cognitive behavioural therapy for non-cardiac chest pain and benign palpitations: A randomised controlled trial. *J Psychosom Res* 70: 117–23.

Kahneman, D. (2011). *Thinking, fast and slow*. New York: Farrar, Straus and Giroux.

Kisely, S.R., Campbell, L.A., Skerritt, P., & Yelland, M.J. (2010). Psychological interventions for symptomatic management of non-specific chest pain in patients with normal coronary anatomy. *The Cochrane Library*. doi: 10.1002/14651858.CD004101.pub3.

Kisley, S.R., Campbell, L.A., Yelland, M.J., & Paydar, A. (2012). Psychological interventions for symptomatic management of non-specific chest pain in patients with normal coronary anatomy (Review). *Cochrane Database Syst Rev* 6: CD004101. 24.

Marks, E.M., Chambers, J.B., Russell, V., & Hunter, M.S. (2014). The rapid access chest pain clinic: Unmet distress and disability. *Q J Med* 107(6): 429–34.

Marks, E.M., Chambers, J.B., Russell, V., & Hunter, M.S. (2016). A novel cognitive behavioural stepped-care intervention for patients with non-cardiac chest pain. *Health Psychol Behav Med* 4(1): 15–28.

Mayou, R., Bryant, B., Forfar, C., & Clark, D. (1994). Non-cardiac chest pain and benign palpitations in the cardiac clinic. *Br Heart J* 2: 548–53.

Padesky, C.A., & Mooney, K.A. (1990). Clinical tip: Presenting the cognitive model to clients. *Int Cogn Ther Newsletter* 6(1): 13–14.

Pampallona, S., Bollini, P., Tibaldi, G., Kupelnick, B., & Munizza, C. (2004). Combined pharmacotherapy and psychological treatment for depression: A systematic review. *Arch Gen Psych* 61(7): 714–19.

Paykel, E.S., Scott, J., Cornwall, P.L., Abbott, R., Crane, C., Pope, M., & Johnson, A.L. (2005). Duration of relapse prevention after cognitive therapy in residual depression: Follow-up of controlled trial. *Psychol Med* 35(1): 59–68.

Petrie, K.J., Muller, J.T., Schirmbeck, F., Donkin, L., Broadbent, E., Ellis, C.J., Gamble, G. & Rief, W. (2007). Effect of providing information about normal test results on patients' reassurance: Randomised controlled trial. *BMJ* 334: 352.

Price, J.R. (2000). Managing physical symptoms: The clinical assessment as treatment. *J Psychosom Res* 48: 1–10.

Salkovskis, P.M. (1991). The importance of behaviour in the maintenance of anxiety and panic: A cognitive account. *Behav Psychother* 19(1): 6–19.

Sanders, D., Bass, C., Mayou, R.A., Goodwin, S., Bryant, B.M., & Forfar, C. (1997). Non-cardiac chest pain: Why was a brief intervention apparently ineffective? *Psychol Med* 27: 1033–40.

Tenkorang, J.N., Fox, K.F., Collier, T.J., & Wood, D.A. (2006). A rapid access cardiology service for chest pain, heart failure and arrhythmias accurately diagnoses cardiac disease and identifies patients at high risk: A prospective cohort study. *Heart* 92: 1084–90.

Turner, J.A., & Romano, J.M. (2001). Cognitive-behavioral therapy for chronic pain. In J.D. Loeser & J.J. Bonica (Eds.), *Bonica's management of pain* (3rd ed., pp. 1751–1758). Philadelphia, PA: Lippincott Williams & Wilkins.

Williams, A.C., Eccleston, C., & Morley, S. (2012). Psychological therapies for the management of chronic pain (excluding headache) in adults. *Cochrane Database Syst Rev* 11: CD007407.

Chapter 7

The biopsychosocial assessment for NCCP

NCCP is caused and maintained by biological and psychosocial factors which vary between individuals. For a biopsychosocial approach to be effective and acceptable, both patient and clinician must work together to develop a shared understanding of all of these factors. This requires very careful assessment. In this chapter, we offer a comprehensive guide to assessing NCCP. This includes suggestions for invitation letters, information sheets and questionnaire measures, which all set the scene for a biopsychosocial approach. The patients in our clinic found this information acceptable. We provide an outline of a semi-structured interview that includes questions to ask and tests that should have been completed by this stage. This assessment is considered to be integral to treatment, as is the written information provided afterwards.

The assessment is designed to be offered to all individuals with NCCP. The treatment in the workbook, however, is designed for individuals with NCCP and mild to moderate psychological distress. If an individual reports either complex medical or psychosocial issues, guided self-help is inappropriate. Instead, the patient should be referred on to specialist care (this could include a clinical psychologist within your clinic). Common complicating factors and how best to manage unexpected scenarios are discussed herein.

Who should do the assessment?

A comprehensive biopsychosocial assessment is the foundation of treatment, and ideally it is conducted jointly by a medical and a psychological specialist (e.g. a consultant cardiologist and a clinical psychologist). A full hour is usually required. Care is taken to emphasize the equal importance of physical and psychosocial factors and how these interact; it can help to interweave the assessment questions asked by each professional as if in a conversation. An experienced cardiologist will provide confidence to the patient in the formulation of NCCP. Paying equal attention to psychosocial and physiological processes reduces concerns about CBT as a psychological approach to a physical symptom. Conducting the combined multidisciplinary clinic in the cardiology department, ideally within the geographical setting of the RACPC, greatly increases the acceptability of the approach and avoids the implied dualism of referring the patient to a separate department of psychology. Over the years, we have run combined cardiology/psychology clinics within a conventional general cardiology outpatient setting with close to 100% uptake and retention.

Adaptions

There are other options for designing a clinic. For example, a cardiac nurse or CBT therapist could work under appropriate supervision from a cardiologist and psychologist. The key point is that cardiac causes for chest pain are reliably and confidently excluded and alternative, plausible and trustworthy biopsychosocial explanations are given. Our clinic accepts referrals (Figure 2.5) after appropriate exclusion of coronary disease. Sometimes there may be NCCP and a cardiac problem, for example, a heart-valve replacement. We also see occasional patients with NCCP after successful revascularization with coronary angioplasty or bypass grafting. In general, 10% of patients report NCCP after coronary bypass grafting (Bruce et al., 2003; Gjeilo et al., 2010). In such cases, you can adapt the treatment, provided there is supervision from a cardiologist.

What you will need before assessment

Expectations and engagement with treatment will depend upon what information the patient has right from the start. Most people with NCCP understandably have a biomedical model of chest pain, so it is important to begin to reshape expectations about a more biopsychosocial approach early on. This involves sending out carefully designed invitation letters and information leaflets (and even a website). An example of a clinic letter appears in Box 7.1. An example of a pre-assessment information leaflet appears in Appendix 1.

BOX 7.1 EXAMPLE INVITATION LETTER

Dear Mrs Jones:

You were recently assessed by the cardiology clinic for persistent chest pain. From the results of this assessment, your doctor felt that your chest pain is unlikely to be caused by heart disease. As there can be many other reasons for ongoing chest pain, your doctor has referred you to our specialist chest pain clinic. We offer assessment and treatment for people with persistent chest pain. Since persistent chest pain can be caused by many different factors, we find it can be very helpful for two team members to meet with you at first. You will be meeting with both Dr Smith (cardiologist) and Dr Williams (psychologist).

We have made an appointment for you on: [date/time/location]

The appointment will last for approximately [1 hour].

We have enclosed a leaflet for you that gives you more information about our clinic and how it may benefit you. We have also included some questionnaires, and we would be grateful if you could complete these and bring them to your appointment; they will help us to ensure you are getting the best treatment. If you would like any more information, please contact me at [phone number].

Yours sincerely,

Mary Jones

Clinical Nurse Specialist

Enc. Information leaflet, questionnaires (PHQ-9, GAD-7, chest pain questions)

A comprehensive biopsychosocial assessment alone can lead to a reduction in negative beliefs about pain and an increase in understanding about the pain (Marks et al., 2016). This can in turn lead to significant improvements in chest pain. Sometimes, no further treatment is required, but a follow-up telephone call can be useful to check that the improvements are not transient and are maintained. In our clinic, most patients tell us that being given a better understanding of chest pain was the single most important factor in their treatment. This means that time has to be spent in exploring each individual's experience of chest pain and how it interacts with (non-cardiac) organic factors, thoughts, behaviours, emotions and other people. The groundwork you do in the first assessment is *critical* to outcome.

Both professionals offer valuable skills. The cardiologist determines organic factors and can arrange medical treatment (medication, further tests or referral onwards). For example, if the pain is associated with acid reflux or postural problems, a purely psychological approach will not alleviate symptoms, whilst medication or physiotherapy might. The psychologist formulates how physical and psychosocial factors interact to maintain chest pain. For example, if chest pain is triggered by stress and over-breathing, then a purely medical approach will probably be ineffective. They can also identify comorbid mental illness, risk issues and the need for specialist psychiatric or psychological input. They can share the biopsychosocial explanation as an alternative hypothesis for NCCP and use a standard CBT model to show how factors interact to influence, trigger and/or maintain pain. This *hypothesis* is then tested using strategies of guided self-help in a person-centred, trial-and-error approach. During treatment, the therapist and patient refine their understanding of chest pain in the light of what they discover over time.

Many clinics may not be able to access clinical psychologists or highly-trained CBT therapists (or receive significant time commitments from a cardiologist). We therefore suggest using the comprehensive assessment protocol developed by our clinic, provided that there is appropriate medical and psychological supervision and full awareness of warning signs and symptoms that indicate a need for further professional input. Such signs include high levels of depression or anxiety (and high questionnaire scores), inconclusive or abnormal test results, or abnormal physical examinations. There should be a nominated cardiologist to offer advice, and usually this will be the person supervising the RACPC. There must be a clear plan for referring to the cardiologist in response to warning signs, although these will be rare (see Box 7.2 later in the chapter).

What you will need during assessment

For the assessment session, ensure that you have the following items (available in Appendices 2 and 3).

- Questionnaire measures/assessment tools and scoring guide (Appendix 2)
- Full biopsychosocial assessment schedule (Appendix 2)
- Information leaflet for after assessment (Appendix 3, handout 1)

Questionnaire measures

Patients should complete brief, standardized questionnaires prior to assessment. These will screen for anxiety (e.g., the GAD-7) and depression (e.g., the PHQ-9) (Kroenke et al., 2001; Spitzer et al., 2006). For useful baseline measures, the patient can complete the following rating scales (Appendix 2):

- Frequency of chest pain
- Chest pain severity and problem ratings
- Cardiac belief ratings

Gathering such information at the initial session can give the clinicians a sense of the patient's experiences, and high scores indicate that additional psychological assessment may be warranted.

Questionnaires repeated every week or less frequently are an excellent way for clinicians and patients to see change. Should you wish to assess changes in other areas, such as quality of life, functioning or activity levels, you could consider additional measures suggested in Table 7.1.

Table 7.1 Screening questionnaires and outcome measures for the chest pain clinic

Chest pain	Frequency (e.g., all the time, several times a day, once per day / week / month). Severity (rated on a 0–10 scale) Interference (average of three items – distress, interference and problem – rated on a 0–10 scale)
Beliefs about chest pain	Belief that chest pain is a heart attack (rated on a 0–10 scale) Belief that chest pain is a sign of serious heart disease (rated on a 0–10 scale)
Depression	Patient Health Questionnaire 9 (PHQ-9) (Kroenke et al., 2001) A total score is calculated from nine items, each rated on a 0–3 scale. Depression severity is indicated by the total score: 0–4 = none; 5–9 = mild; 10–14 = moderate; 15–19 = moderately severe; 20–27 = severe depression. Any person scoring 10 or more can be regarded as suffering from clinically significant symptoms of depression.
Anxiety	Generalized Anxiety Disorder Scale 7 (GAD-7) (Spitzer et al., 2006) A total score is calculated from seen items, each rated on a 0–3 scale. Anxiety severity is indicated by the total score: 0–5 = mild; 6–10 = moderate; 11–15 = moderately severe; 16–21 = severe anxiety. Any person scoring 8 or more can be regarded as suffering from clinically significant symptoms of anxiety.
Activity	Frequency of avoiding activity and engaging in exercise (Jonsbu et al., 2011) You could consider using this as an additional measure to assess the degree to which an individual avoids exercise because of their chest pain.
Impact on daily life	Work and Social Adjustment Scale (WSAS) (Mundt et al., 2002). You could consider using this as an additional measure to assess the impact of chest pain and associated symptoms on a person's functioning.
Illness perceptions	Brief Illness Perceptions Questionnaire (BIPQ) (Broadbent et al., 2006). You could use this additional measure to assess people's perception of chest pain and its impact.

How to conduct the assessment

To help identify what questions will be asked by each clinician, we have divided our explanation of the assessment process into medical and psychosocial sections. Each section also lists indicators for further care to clarify when an individual may need more assessment or intervention than is offered here.

In practise, we recommend that the medical and psychosocial questions be interwoven. The factors relevant to the patient can be discussed in terms of the biopsychosocial model. Once the assessment is complete, we suggest that the patient leave the room for a short break while the two professionals agree on the factors affecting the patient and the appropriate treatment plan. When the patient returns, the biopsychosocial explanation and treatment recommendations are given, along with written information to take home. The patient needs to have an opportunity to offer their own perspective on these conclusions and identify how treatment can fit with their lifestyle and preferences.

For a summary overview of the questions to follow as you conduct the biopsychosocial assessment, we recommend using the Full Biopsychosocial Assessment Schedule in Appendix 2.

Introducing the assessment

The patient may not understand why they are meeting with two clinicians, so you may wish to begin by explaining who each person is and what their different areas of expertise are. You can find out what the patient thought of the information leaflet and use this to reinforce that chest pain is common, benign and usually caused by a range of physical and psychosocial factors. You may wish to explain that in addition to asking about chest pain, you will also explore the person's life and general health. Also explain that the cardiologist (or other medical practitioner) will conduct a brief physical examination.

Since the assessment could touch upon sensitive issues, you may wish to make explicit the limits of confidentiality and other service-specific issues. When risk factors are identified, or if you feel that onward referral is required, this will be much easier to manage if you have a clear prior agreement about what will happen with this information (such as sharing it with the GP).

Medical assessment

The medical history is extended in detail so that you have a full description of chest pain characteristics (including onset, duration, nature, radiation, relieving factors, frequency and the presence of extra-cardiac symptoms). The medical assessment is designed to uncover alternative mechanisms for chest pain, as described in Chapter 3. Table 7.2 gives a summary.

Table 7.2 Summary of medical assessment

A description of the chest pain

The Guy's chest pain questionnaire
Typicality score 0–3: 0 = non-cardiac, 1–2 = atypical, 3 = typical

	Score 1 if:	*Score 0 if:*
1 If you have 10 pains (or tightness or breathlessness) in a row, how many occur on exercise?	10	0–9
2 How many occur at rest?	0–1	2–10
3 How long does the pain last?	≤5 min	>5 min

Other chest pain questions
Does it occur during or after exercise? Does it make you stop or slow down?
What is the frequency and duration?
Site and radiation? Does it vary in position?
What were you doing before or during the first pain episode?

Breathlessness
Is there air hunger?
Is there breathlessness especially during eating or talking?
Does the patient report sighing, gasping, throat clearing, globus?
Does the patient report pins and needles around the mouth or fingers (on the right or left side)?
Is there hyperacusis or photophobia (sensitivity to sound or light – e.g. wearing dark glasses with no opthalmological need)?

Gastrointestinal
Is there acid reflux, water brash or dysphagia?
Does the pain occur after food, with particular types of food or when lying or bending?
Is the pain relieved by antacids, fluids or eating?
Are there symptoms of irritable bowel (variable stool consistency, mucus, precipitancy, bloating, flatulence)?

Musculoskeletal
Is there morning stiffness?
Does the pain happen with moving the arms, neck or other joints?

Points in the examination
Evidence of a breathing abnormality
Thoracic respiratory pattern
Sighing
Throat clearing
Localized chest wall tenderness
Breath-holding time reduced (<20 sec) (Does this induce the usual pain?)
Voluntary overbreathing at rest for 60 seconds (Does this induce the usual pain?)

Evidence of a musculoskeletal abnormality
Springing the spine
Movement of neck
Crepitus and reduced mobility at shoulder
Localized joint tenderness
Physical exam – evidence of a breathing abnormality

Further investigation may sometimes be necessary (Chapter 5) if cardiac disease has not been adequately excluded. Box 7.2 highlights what indicators for further medical assessment to look out for. More rarely, you may feel that specific tests for non-cardiac causes of chest pain are needed. It is important to remember that negative tests without a proper explanation may fail to reassure your patient, whilst pursuing tests may reinforce the unhelpful idea that there is an underlying organic abnormality.

BOX 7.2 INDICATORS FOR FURTHER ASSESSMENT AND CARE EMERGING FROM THE MEDICAL ASSESSMENT

New symptoms can develop or the nature of symptoms can appear to change during assessment. Consider asking for further medical advice in the following scenarios.

Before starting treatment

1 Coronary disease is not adequately excluded: No anatomical (coronary angiography) or functional (e.g. stress echocardiogram) cardiac test despite:

- Chest pain occurring reproducibly on exertion or
- Atypical pain with numerous coronary risk factors (e.g. age > 50, smoking, diabetes, family history, hypertension, dyslipidaemia).

2 Coronary disease is present or possible (i.e. cardiac tests positive or equivocal, unless the cardiologist has proven that this is no longer symptomatic).
3 Symptoms suggesting significant organic disease:

- Blood loss
- Weight loss
- Food seems to stick in the oesophagus.

4 There are psychiatric abnormalities.

During treatment

There is a change in the chest pain characteristics, especially if it becomes reproducibly related to exertion.

Psychosocial assessment

Questions focus on associations between chest pain and life changes, thoughts and beliefs, emotions, behaviours and the patient's social environment. Life stressors are identified and linked to chest pain. Positive and protective factors are included. All of the information is used to develop an individualized CBT model of NCCP (see Chapter 5) known as the patient's chest pain cycle (Figure 7.1). The chest pain cycle is a diagrammatic summary of assessment that forms the basis of treatment. Screening for comorbidities (depression and anxiety) is important, to determine suitability for inclusion in your clinic. Exploring the patient's goals for the future is needed to support treatment planning.

Chest pain cycle questions

It helps to focus your early questions on chest pain, possibly by asking about the first episode, as this can highlight triggers, interpretations and reactions. Many people with NCCP have had stressful life events before

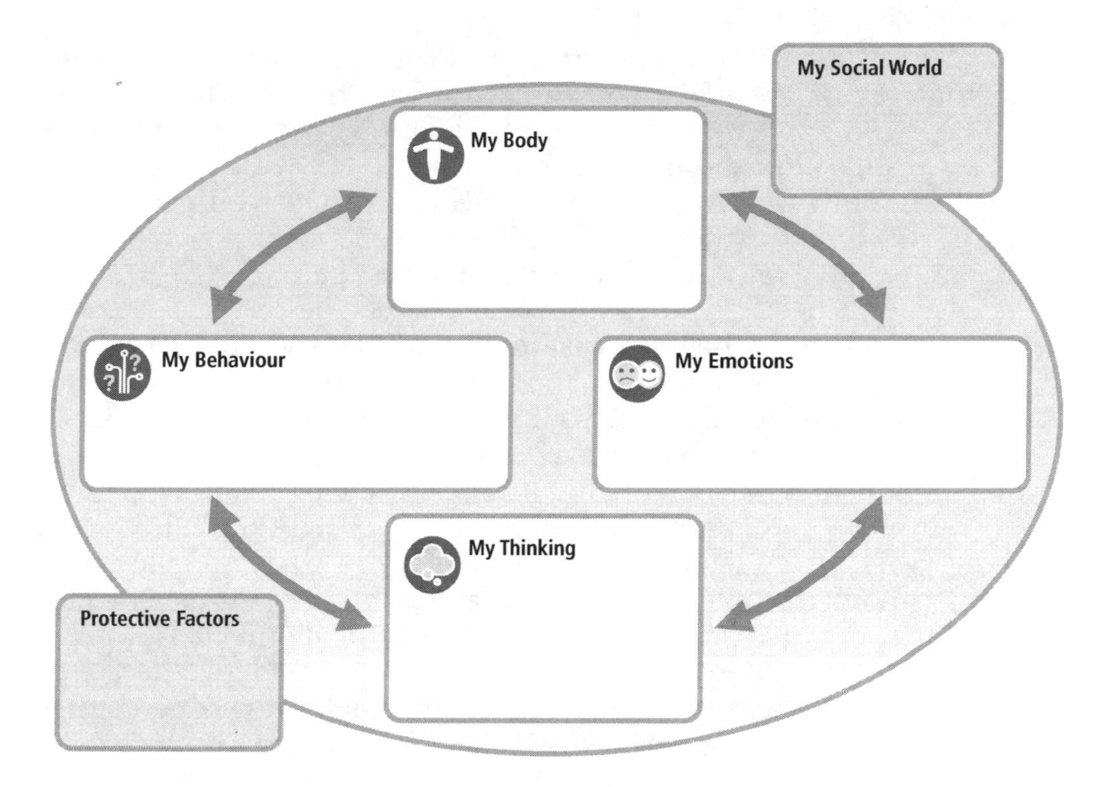

Figure 7.1 The chest pain cycle

Each section of this chest pain cycle can be completed using the specific body sensations, thoughts, emotions, behaviours, social world and protective factors that emerge during assessment and throughout treatment.

or around the time of their first episode, although not all will have recognized this. Few patients will have had time to talk about the profound impact of chest pain with a professional, so offering them this time to talk can forge strong therapeutic rapport. It can help to use gentle prompts to explore the impact of chest pain on different life domains. You may like to note down the specific words used by the patient to reflect back to them later on.

Develop the chest pain cycle by asking about specific factors in turn. Find out what the patient thinks, feels, senses and does and how their social world is relevant when NCCP occurs. Details are often recalled more precisely when a recent, typical episode of chest pain is recounted. Since NCCP can have a broad impact on life, it is valuable to find out what happens between episodes. For example, immediate fears during chest pain ("I'm going to die!") may be followed by more chronic worry after it stops ("My kids won't survive without me"; "It might come back any minute"). Gentle exploration of both immediate and ongoing reactions to chest pain can indicate how chest pain produces immediate and sustained distress.

The following questions may help:

1 Can you remember a recent episode of chest pain that was quite representative for you? Where were you? What were you doing? Was anything else happening? Was anyone else there?

2 *Thoughts*: What went through your mind? Did you have any images in your mind? What did you think was causing it? What did you think would happen? Did you think something bad might happen? Did you still think about it afterwards?
3 *Emotions*: How did you feel about chest pain? Did you get scared, anxious, angry, frustrated or sad? How do you feel afterwards? How do you feel generally about your life and chest pain?
4 *Behaviours*: What did you do when you first felt chest pain? For example, did you stop what you were doing, rest or seek help? Did you focus on the chest pain or try to ignore it? Is this what you usually do? Have you changed what you used to do in your daily life since getting chest pain? In what way?
5 *Body sensations:* Did you notice anything else changing or happening in your body, for example, feeling breathless or lightheaded?
6 *Social world*: How did other people react? Is this what normally happens? Do other people understand what is happening? Is anyone particularly supportive or unsupportive of you at the moment? How have health professionals reacted to your chest pain? How did this affect you?
7 *Positive and protective factors*: Did anything help you cope at that point? Does anything ever help? Is there anything in your life right now about which you feel positive What helps you to keep going despite chest pain?

Goals for treatment

Patient goals and hopes for the future affect their motivation, engagement and treatment success. Usually the main goal is to find a cure, that is, to stop or reduce pain. As NCCP may not always be cured, it is essential to find out what else is important to the individual, in particular, how chest pain limits their life. So, even if NCCP persists, treatment is effective if the patient can minimize their limitations to live well despite the pain. You can find out what would be different in their life if chest pain were no longer an issue. Concrete examples are easier to work with, so it helps to identify what someone might be doing differently if NCCP were not an issue or what they did before NCCP. Goal-setting is discussed in more detail in session 1 of the workbook.

Psychosocial stressors

As discussed in Chapter 5, stress is common in NCCP, but it may not be easy for patients to recognize or disclose. General queries about possible sources stress, followed up by exploring associations with chest pain, can be helpful. Chest pain itself is a stressor. Discussions are facilitated if stress is normalized as a universal experience that is frequently reported by other people. Common stressors include bereavement, relational conflict, housing issues, legal problems, financial worries, unemployment, workplace bullying and so on.

Many psychosocial stressors will be adequately tackled using the stress management and problem-solving strategies in the guided self-help treatment. If the treating clinician has additional therapeutic skills and experience, they can adapt the guided self-help to manage more specific issues. For example, our clinical psychologist included a session of supportive bereavement counselling for a patient who was recently bereaved and on assertiveness skills for a patient with work problems. Otherwise, you can refer the patient to appropriate services (see Section 3 of the book for specific recommendations.

Screening for psychiatric comorbidities

Psychiatric comorbidities are common in NCCP, and some can even directly cause chest pain (particularly if panic attacks are part of the presentation). This does not automatically preclude treatment, and treatment for NCCP has been found to lead to substantial reductions in both depression and anxiety. However, unless your clinic has access to an experienced mental health practitioner, it is not appropriate to offer treatment for NCCP to patients with significant psychiatric comorbidities. If assessment indicates a comorbid mental health disorder, we strongly recommend that the individual is referred for further psychological or psychiatric assessment.

Anxiety and depression

These are the most common psychiatric comorbidities in NCCP, specifically panic disorder and health anxiety. People may also report symptoms of post-traumatic stress disorder (PTSD), obsessive compulsive disorder (OCD), psychosis or other severe mental illness. Identifying and diagnosing these problems requires specific psychiatric or psychological training. However, you can use screening questionnaires to indicate whether an individual may have psychological distress at a level warranting further care. The PHQ-9 assesses depression, and a score of 20 or more on the PHQ-9 indicates severe depression. The GAD-7 assesses anxiety, and a score of 16 or more on the GAD-7 indicates severe anxiety. Collecting these questionnaires before assessment will give you an opportunity to recognize which patients may need more support than your clinic can offer.

Panic disorder

The symptoms of a panic attack share similarities with NCCP, and for many patients the anxiety associated with chest pain can cause panic attacks. A panic attack is an abrupt surge of intense fear or discomfort occurring from a calm or an anxious state, peaking in minutes, during which four or more of the following symptoms occur:

> Palpitations, pounding heart, or accelerated heart rate; sweating; trembling or shaking; sensations of shortness of breath or smothering; feeling of choking; chest pain or discomfort; nausea or abdominal distress; feeling dizzy, unsteady, lightheaded, or faint; chills or heat sensations; numbness or tingling sensations; feelings of unreality; feelings of being detached from oneself; fear of losing control or going crazy; fear of dying.
>
> *The Diagnositic and Statistical Manual of Mental Diseases*, 5th Edition

Panic disorder is diagnosed when attacks are frequent, there is significant worry about the consequences of the attacks and there are major behavioural changes. If the patient reports panic attacks occurring outside of NCCP episodes, it is more appropriate to refer them on for further assessment and care.

Health anxiety

Symptoms include high levels of anxiety about health when somatic symptoms are not present or a preoccupation that one has a serious illness based on the misinterpretation of bodily sensations and despite appropriate medical evaluation and reassurance. There is a clear overlap with NCCP, but health anxiety will usually include additional worry about other (sometimes multiple) aspects of health. Guided self-help for NCCP may be of benefit but will probably be less effective in the context of health anxiety. You may find that anxiety remains high even after treatment, with worry moving on to another aspect of health, and this may warrant referral on for further care.

Other mental health problems

Patients with NCCP may sometimes report other mental health problems. In our clinic, a few patients presented with PTSD, OCD and psychosis. A clinical psychologist can extend assessment to identify these issues. Without a mental health professional, assessment will have to depend on the judicious use of screening questionnaires to identify the presence of heightened psychological distress. It may also be worth contacting the GP for further information if you are concerned or if the patient reports engagement with a mental health service.

Managing complex psychosocial issues

It is still possible to offer treatment for NCCP in the context of relatively mild comorbid mental health problems and social stressors. In cases of mild to moderate depression, the treatment approach described here is suitable, particularly if appropriate supervision is available or a trained mental health professional is delivering treatment. However, more severe issues require more specialist psychological/psychiatric care, and if this is not available in your service, it is best practice to refer on for further care. This may include:

- Referral back to the GP. Consider writing back to the GP a summary of your assessment and need for these other issues to be managed before NCCP treatment can be offered.
- Referral to psychiatric liaison.
- Referral to local psychological therapy services (the UK Improving Access to Psychological Therapies [IAPT] initiative – see Section 3).

Risk

Patients sometimes report risk of harm to self (e.g. suicidal ideation or past suicide attempts, substance misuse or deliberate self-harm), risk of harm from others (e.g. domestic violence or risk of exploitation) or risk of harm to others (e.g. violent or aggressive behaviour). We advise that risk is assessed and managed in line with your standard clinical protocols. This will probably involve discussion with the GP and sometimes the safeguarding team. Patients may be under the care of another service, in which case careful liaison will confirm whether it is appropriate for the patient to receive your treatment for NCCP.

Indicators for further care that may emerge from the psychosocial assessment and screening questionnaires are summarized in Box 7.3, and it is worth being familiar with these before beginning an assessment.

BOX 7.3 INDICATORS FOR FURTHER ASSESSMENT AND CARE EMERGING FROM THE PSYCHOSOCIAL ASSESSMENT AND SCREENING QUESTIONNAIRES

If a qualified mental health practitioner is conducting the assessment, it can be extended to find out more about the following issues. If the assessment is conducted by someone without training in psychological assessment, then if any of the following issues arise, the patient should be referred on for further assessment and care.

continued

Severe depression

- Severe score on PHQ-9 questionnaire (total score of 20–27).
- Reported risk of self-harm or suicidal ideation (including a positive response to question 9 on PHQ-9).

Severe anxiety disorders

- Severe score on GAD-7 questionnaire (total score of 16–21).
- Panic disorder: repeated panic attacks, independent of chest pain.
- Health anxiety: significant worry about aspects of their health *other than* chest pain, despite medical reassurance.

Risk issues

- Reported risk of harming themselves: current or recent suicidal ideation, suicide attempts or self-harm, or substance misuse (alcohol or drug use).
- Reported risk of harm from another person: abuse, domestic violence, exploitation.
- Reported risk of harming others: recent acts of violence or aggression, or unable to care for vulnerable dependents.

Currently receiving psychological/psychiatric treatment elsewhere

- This need not automatically preclude treatment, but liaison with the GP and psychologist/psychiatrist is advised, with the patient's consent.

Examples of working with NCCP and more complex presentations

The following cases based on patients who attended our clinic offer examples of how it is possible to treat NCCP symptoms directly even if the overall presentation includes additional and more complex psychosocial issues:

- CBT for patients with PTSD and associated panic attacks was tailored to include psychoeducation about PTSD and panic.
- Treatment for a patients with more severe and enduring mental health problems who were already supported by psychologists in the local mental health team can be delivered as a focused intervention, following the guided self-help protocol.
- Patients with health anxiety, panic disorder or OCD can complete an adapted treatment for NCCP by including additional CBT elements such as disorder-specific psychoeducation and cognitive behavioural strategies.

In these cases, a positive outcome from the NCCP intervention can provide a greater understanding about the roles of thoughts, emotions and physical sensations in emotional distress, and this often leads to improved well-being and better engagement with other services.

Table 7.3 offers an overview of the questions that need to be asked as part of the psychosocial focus of the assessment, following which you should have gathered sufficient information to complete the chest pain cycle.

Table 7.3 Summary of psychosocial assessment

Initial chest pain
When did you first have chest pain? What happened?
What else was happening in your life at this time?
Chest pain sometimes starts during or after a stressful time; is this true for you?
Had you ever had chest pain before this?
Impact
How has chest pain affected your life as a whole?
Effect on your quality of life, relationships, work, activity, family life?
CBT chest pain cycle
Tell me about a recent, typical episode of chest pain
Thoughts
What went through your mind? What did you think was happening or would happen?
Emotions
How did you feel? How do you feel about chest pain more generally?
Behaviour
What did you do? Did you focus on it? Did you avoid or do things differently because you were having chest pain? How do you do this and why?
Sensations
Did you notice other body sensations? Is this typical?
Other people
How did other people react? Is this typical? Do people treat you differently because of chest pain now? How does this affect you?
Protective factors
What positive things are happening in your life right now? What helps you to keep going? What helps you cope with chest pain?
What are your goals and hopes for treatment
Psychiatric Screening
Depression
How is your mood? Do you feel down? Is this unusual? Do you ever have thoughts about harming yourself?
Check PHQ-9: scores > 10 indicate depression; scores > 20 indicate severe depression (refer for further care).
Anxiety
Do you get anxious a lot? Do you worry about things a lot? Do you have problems with sleep or feeling tired?
Check GAD-7: scores > 7 indicate anxiety; scores >15 indicate severe anxiety (refer for further care).
Panic
Do you get panic attacks? Do they happen with chest pain? What causes them? Do they ever happen without chest pain occurring?

continued

Table 7.3 (Continued)

Health anxiety
Other than chest pain, do you tend to worry about other aspects of your health?
Other
Have you ever been diagnosed with a mental health problem either now or in the past?
Are you currently receiving support for your well-being at the moment, for example from a counsellor, psychologist or psychiatrist? What is this and where is it? May I have your consent to liaise with this clinician?
Stress
In today's world, most of us have something difficult or stressful in our lives. Is there anything that you are finding stressful now or recently?
Is there anything else that you have not yet mentioned, such as problems at work, in relationships or with finances, housing, recent losses or changes?

Completing the individual chest pain cycle

Pertinent factors from assessment are used to draw out the individualized CBT chest pain cycle for the patient, and these should be written down during assessment. Ideally you will have a few minutes when the patient leaves the room to discuss the chest pain cycle with your colleague, so you can agree how it will be completed. A blank chest pain cycle is available in Figure 7.1. Once completed, the patient returns and together you can work through the diagram and explain how it fits what they have told you.

Triggers: You may like to begin with the most obvious chest pain trigger. For example, if stress clearly causes NCCP, you could start at the emotions box. If muscle strain from bad posture is a more obvious trigger, you could start at the body box.

Body: This box addresses underlying medical or physical cause for chest pain, as well as sensations that co-occur with chest pain.

Thoughts: This box addresses thoughts and fears about chest pain (especially beliefs about causes and consequences). Include thoughts occurring with chest pain and those that happen between episodes.

Emotions: This addresses emotions that occur before, during and after chest pain episodes. Try to check that the emotions reported make sense and fit with the thoughts. If the patient struggles to identify the emotion, you could offer a few suggestions (e.g. "You thought that you were having a heart attack, I could imagine that might have made you feel scared or worried or something similar? Was that the case?").

Behaviours: This addresses immediate reactions to chest pain as well as behaviours occurring between episodes (possibly to avoid or reduce pain) and before episodes (potential triggers).

Social world: This addresses typical reactions to chest pain by other people, both immediately and in the longer term.

Protective and positive factors: These are techniques that enhance coping and positive aspects in the patient's life.

Following the assessment: what to do next

Once the chest pain cycle has been completed and shared with the patient, you can decide on the treatment approach. This includes appropriate medical treatment. Patients with NCCP and with no indicators for further care are suitable for the guided self-help approach outlined in the workbook in Section 2 of this book. We offer the first treatment session 2 weeks after assessment so the patient has time to think about our discussions and commence any medication.

Meanwhile, we give the patient written information to take home that reiterates the biopsychosocial model of NCCP and other helpful information. This is available in Appendix 3 as Handout 1. For patients with more complex presentations, time should be spent agreeing on an referral pathway. Handout 1 should only be given to those patients with clear NCCP who are suitable for this treatment approach.

Case study: developing an individual chest pain cycle for Suzie

Suzie was a 39-year-old woman with persistent NCCP. The issues arising from her assessment are summarized. This is followed by a diagrammatic representation of the biopsychosocial model of her chest pain (her individualized chest pain cycle, Figure 7.2).

Suzie's first chest pain episode began a few minutes after an argument with a work colleague. She felt hot and sweaty, she couldn't catch her breath and felt light-headed. Her immediate thought was that this was a heart attack. She was very scared. A colleague saw her looking ill and called an ambulance. At the hospital she had lots of tests, including an angiogram and a treadmill test. However, the doctors told her that nothing was wrong, and she was discharged. Suzie believed that the doctors had missed something, because she continued to have chest pain several times a week. She decided to research it on the Internet, which made her even more worried, because she learnt about how chest pain might be a sign of dangerous heart disease.

Suzie felt responsible for monitoring her chest for any signs of a heart problem. She would pay attention to her heart rate and chest sensations, particularly when exercising. She began to notice that sensations in her chest changed all the time and that her heart would beat faster when she exercised or felt stressed. Her chest pains began to happen more often. She thought that stress and exercising too much were putting her in danger, so she stopped doing anything active, and whenever her heart began to beat faster, she would stop and rest. She felt unable to do certain household chores, stopped socializing and even reduced her working hours. Her family was worried and encouraged Suzie to take more rest. As a result, she was often alone at home, and she would sit and think about how she couldn't cope with chest pain, which made her feel very sad. Her GP referred her to the RACPC for more tests, all of which were still normal. At this point, she was referred to our biopsychosocial chest pain clinic, where the psychologist and cardiologist assessed her.

Suzie's medical assessment

A thoracic breathing style was identified. Suzie was breathless when talking on the telephone and her breath-holding time was only 5 seconds. Voluntary overbreathing induced chest pain within 20 seconds. The physical examination found localized tenderness around the shoulders, and Suzie described how the tenderness increased when she felt tense and stressed.

Information for Suzie's chest pain cycle

Suzie's first chest pain episode occurred after interpersonal conflict, in the context of general work-related stress. It was associated with tension and overbreathing. The overbreathing test in the assessment session had already triggered chest pain, so this physical factor offered a good starting point for the chest pain cycle.

Body: Chest pain, heart rate increased, breathlessness, light-headed. Underlying physical cause identified as a thoracic breathing pattern and muscle tension which increases with stress.

Thoughts: I'm having a heart attack; Chest pain is dangerous; I'm going to die; I need to protect my heart by resting; I can't cope; The doctors have missed something; I'm a burden on my family.

Emotions: Fear and terror when chest pain occurs. Anxiety, stress and sadness between episodes (increasing over time).

Behaviours: When chest pain occurs, lie down and sometimes call an ambulance, the GP or go to hospital. More generally, rest if any sensations are noticed in the chest. Avoid activity or exercise, reduce working hours, research information on the Internet and focus attention on the chest.

Social world: Stress at work. Family very concerned about Suzie's health. Unclear messages from hospital doctors, who have not explained what is causing the chest pain. Isolation, reduced employment, no longer engaging in many positive activities.

Protective and positive factors: Supportive family members who want to help. Suzie feels very motivated to find a way to change things and to use any strategies available to her. She recognizes the link between stress and chest pain.

This information was used to develop Suzie's chest pain cycle, elucidating each factor and showing important interactions between them (Figure 7.2).

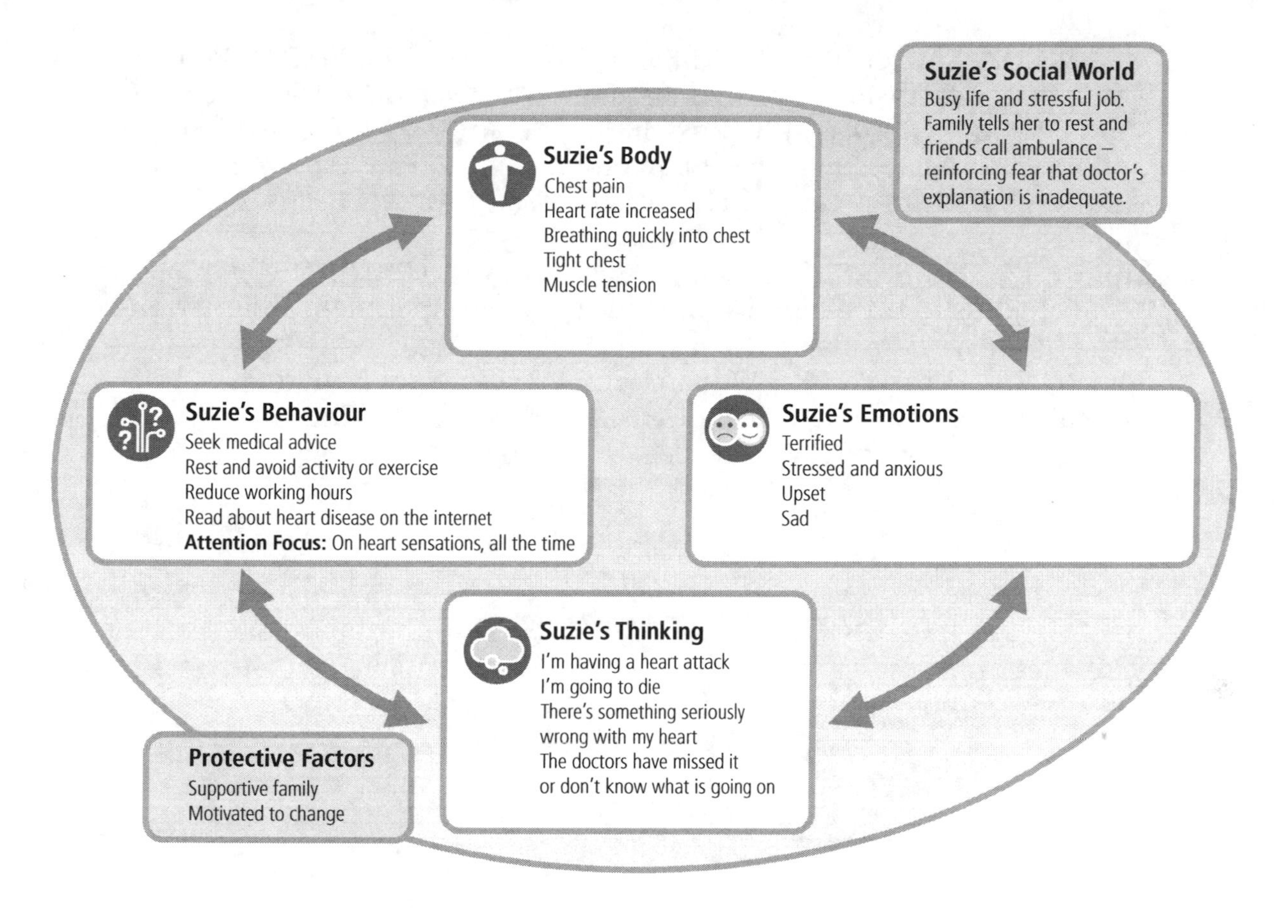

Figure 7.2 Suzie's chest pain cycle

References

American Psychiatric Association (2013). *Diagnostic and Statistical Manual of Mental Disorders* (5th Edition). Washington, DC: Author.

Broadbent, E., Petrie, K.J., Maina, J., & Weinman, J. (2006). The brief illness perception questionnaire. *J Psychosom Res* 60: 631–7.

Bruce, J., Drury, N., Poobalan, A.S., Jeffrey, R.R., Smith, W.C.S., & Chambers, W.A. (2003). The prevalence of chronic chest and leg pain following cardiac surgery: A historical cohort study. *Pain* 104: 265–73.

Chambers, J.B., Marks, E.M., Russell, V., & Hunter, M.S. (2014). A multidisciplinary, biopsychosocial treatment for non-cardiac chest pain. *Int J Clin Pract*. doi:10.1111/ijcp.12533

Gjeilo, K.H., Klepstad, P., Wahba, A., Lydersen, S., & Stenseth, R. (2010). Chronic pain after cardiac surgery: A prospective study. *Acta Anaesthesiol Scan* 54: 70–8.

Jonsbu, E., Dammen, T., Morken, G., Moum, T., & Martinsen, E.W. (2011). Short-term cognitive behavioural therapy for non-cardiac chest pain and benign palpitations: A randomized controlled trial. *J Psychosom Res* 70: 117–23.

Kroenke, K., Spitzer, R.L., & Williams, J.B. (2001). The PHQ-9: Validity of a brief depression severity measure. *J Gen Intern Med* 16(9): 606–13.

Marks, E.M., Chambers, J.B., Russell, V., & Hunter, M.S. (2016). A novel biopsychosocial, cognitive behavioural, stepped care intervention for patients with non-cardiac chest pain. *Health Psychol Behav Med* 4(1): 15–28.

Mundt, J.C., Marks, I.M., Shear, K., & Greist, J.H. (2002). The work and social adjustment scale: A simple measure of impairment in functioning. *Br J Psychiatry* 180: 461–4.

Spitzer, R.L., Kroenke, K., Williams, J.B.W., & Lowe, B. (2006). A brief measure for assessing Generalized Anxiety Disorder: The GAD-7. *Arch Intern Med* 166: 1092–7.

Section 2

The workbook

How to use the workbook

This workbook provides a treatment manual for delivering guided self-help (low-intensity CBT) to people with NCCP. The treatment is only suitable for individuals who have had a full assessment and have satisfactorily been found to have chest pain that is not of cardiac origin. It is not appropriate for patients with underlying cardiac problems or complex psychosocial issues requiring intensive or specialist care.

The workbook rests on the assumption the patient has been appropriately assessed, preferably using the methods described in Chapter 7, by a cardiologist and a psychologist (or a nurse who has received training in this approach). After this, the patient should have been provided with handout 1 in Appendix 3. The guided self-help can then be offered by the same psychologist or nurse. The advantage of having completed a joint assessment is that it sets the scene for biopsychosocial work. The patient will benefit from the wealth of expertise offered and can feel assured that no important issues have been missed.

Treatment cannot begin unless there is reasonable medical certainty that coronary disease has been excluded (see Chapter 2) and alternative factors likely to be causing and maintaining NCCP have been identified. Treatment should also rest upon the individualized chest pain cycle created out of assessment, which can be shared with the patient immediately. If the clinician guiding the self-help is not involved in the assessment process, then it is essential that they have a copy of the individual's chest pain cycle and any other relevant information.

Who should offer treatment?

The workbook has been designed by clinical psychologists, cardiologists and cardiac nurses. It offers a detailed, session-by-session guide with handouts and audio guides to give to the patient. The workbook does not train the clinician to become a CBT practitioner or to offer high-intensity CBT. It is a standardized intervention grounded in CBT principles, offering treatment only at the level of guided self-help. It should be delivered by a health care professional with training in CBT and access to ongoing CBT supervision, such as nurse specialists, primary care staff or low-intensity CBT workers. In our clinic, cardiac nurses with no prior experience in CBT initially receive approximately 3 days of training from our clinical psychologist. Training focuses on understanding the CBT stance of collaboration with the patient and specific instruction on how to enable patients to learn and use the specific strategies and ideas in the workbook. This initial training stage is followed by the nurse observing the psychologist using the workbook, then the psychologist observing the nurse delivering each session of the workbook. After this, there should be fortnightly clinical supervision.

This manual is based on the principles of CBT and biopsychosocial approaches to NCCP, so some knowledge and skills in these areas is advantageous, particularly if there is no access to specific training. In offering treatment, we advise adhering to the competencies for practitioners, described by Improving Access to Psychological Therapies (IAPT) (Rimes et al., 2014). This sits within the stepped care model described in Chapter 7 (Espie, 2009).

The workbook is designed to be closely followed in order to deliver low-intensity CBT. However, experienced CBT therapists may find it a helpful clinical tool that will support the delivery of high-intensity CBT in more complex cases:

- *Low-intensity CBT using the workbook:* The workbook is a comprehensive manualized treatment plan that is appropriate only for patients with NCCP and without complex or severe psychosocial issues. It is appropriate for patients with mild anxiety and/or depression. As such, the workbook offers treatment at levels 1 and 2 of the stepped care pyramid, and it is best delivered by practitioners with training in CBT, such as cardiac nurses or psychological well-being practitioners with appropriate clinical supervision. Low-intensity work is designed to meet a high volume of individuals so sessions can be limited to 30 minutes.
- *High-intensity CBT in addition to the workbook:* The workbook alone is not sufficient for patients with NCCP and complex psychosocial problems, including moderate to severe depression or anxiety disorders, risk issues and complex social problems. Such patients will require more support with an experienced clinician fully trained in CBT. This includes practitioners meeting criteria for levels 3 and 4 for stepped care, such as clinical psychologists, counselling psychologists and CBT therapists. It is possible to base high-intensity CBT for NCCP on the workbook, as the clinical psychologist in our clinic does. However, the clinician must be able to respond to complex comorbidities by adapting the treatment as necessary. If your clinic does not have access to a practitioner trained to deliver high intensity CBT, then the patient should not be offered guided self-help, but should instead be referred for further psychological care. High-intensity CBT for NCCP tends to involve longer sessions of 50 minutes.

The workbook describes how to deliver a six-session, low-intensity CBT intervention. Sessions can be weekly or fortnightly. There are six sections in the workbook (one per session). We recommend completing the entire workbook in the order suggested. Sometimes you may need to omit a chapter if it is not relevant to an individual or if someone has already responded well to therapy and does not require the full six sessions. Although low-intensity CBT usually involves 30 minute appointments, clinicians new to this approach may prefer to offer 50 minutes at first.

Adapting the workbook

As we have discussed, NCCP is a diagnosis of exclusion, so patients vary considerably in their presentations and needs. There will be a range of responses to the stepped care approach, and some patients will require more input than others. Some examples of this happening in our clinic are shown next.

Example 1: a case of assessment alone being adequate

Paul, 35, first had chest pain 4 months ago. Since it came after a large celebration involving a lot of eating and drinking, Paul thought it was just indigestion, so he ignored it. When he then told his wife, she was more concerned and persuaded him to go to the emergency department at the local hospital. Paul was quickly discharged after being told that his heart was fine. He felt confused, however, because he didn't understand why he needed so many tests if he was fine. He began to worry about the pain more and more. After finishing assessment, he told us that it had been very helpful to understand what was happening, and he was prescribed Lanzoprazole (a proton pump inhibitor) because his symptoms indicated gastro-oesophageal reflux. By session 1, he had been taking Lanzoprazole for 2 weeks, and he had experienced immediate reduction in his chest pain. He quickly stopped worrying about chest pain and decided that he didn't need any more help. We agreed to use the time in session 1 to review his chest pain cycle and summarize how this had helped. Paul had an option to contact us over the next 6 weeks if he wanted more support. He did not require further help and his chest pain did not recur.

Example 2: a case where fewer CBT sessions were needed

Sarah, 62, had been having chest pain for about a year. She was worried that it could be related to her heart, since her father and elder brother had both died from a myocardial infarction in their early 60s. The assessment had identified how her chest pain was probably related to high levels of stress from her busy life, causing muscular tension and chest breathing, and this had led to increasing negative thoughts about her heart with concomitant anxiety. Sarah agreed that she had never learnt how to relax properly and that she had always put great demands on herself. As a result, she was still very active, but now whenever she had pain, she would stop and rest. Sarah practised the breathing and relaxation exercises regularly (from sessions 2 and 3) and began to make more time for herself. By session 4, her chest pain was less severe, she had stopped worrying about her heart and she no longer discontinued activity in response to chest pain. She told us that treatment had been so successful that she didn't need to have any more sessions. We therefore did not offer her sessions 4 and 5, but spent her final session ensuring that her maintenance plan (see session 6) explicitly identified how helpful thoughts and behaviours had played a role in her recovery.

What to do when there is immediate improvement and treatment seems unnecessary

Some people with NCCP report immediate improvement after assessment, particularly if medication has stopped the symptoms (e.g. of gastric reflux). We audited the results of our clinic and found that this happened in about 5% of people. Most benefitted from some further support, although not all needed to complete all six sessions.

At follow up, we asked our patients to identify the three most helpful parts of treatment, and these were:

1 Abdominal breathing (even if thoracic breathing patterns had *not* been identified at assessment)
2 Worrying less about pain
3 Improved understanding about pain

We found that the average number of sessions, including assessment, was four, showing how treatment can be successful in fewer than six sessions. However, we offer the full six sessions of treatment here because different patients will benefit from different treatment. If you do decide to offer fewer sessions, you will need to exercise clinical judgement when deciding which sessions can be omitted. For example, patients who do not avoid activity may not need a session focused on ways to increase activity, and patients with low levels of stress may not need a session focused on stress management.

Patients who show immediate or rapid improvement will still benefit from a review session a few weeks later, and this will allow you to ensure that benefits are sustained over time and help the patient to remember what parts of treatment are useful (should they relapse). A brief telephone follow up can be sufficient.

The structure of the workbook

The workbook begins with a recap of the patient's individual chest pain cycle, that is, how biological, psychological and social factors interact and influence their chest pain. Patient-centred care is supported if the therapist has the individual's chest pain cycle, even if they did not conduct the assessment. For ease of description, we will be using the term NCCP throughout the workbook. However, it is better when working with patients to use a term such as *persistent* or *chronic chest pain,* which may be more acceptable (and which is not associated with the heart).

Session 1 reinforces the biopsychosocial understanding of NCCP and alternative explanations for chest pain that are not associated with serious disease. It identifies values-based goals for the patient to work towards. This shared understanding is the ground upon which your collaborative relationship and treatment will stand.

Session 2 looks at how breathing styles can affect chest pain and teaches the patient how to use abdominal, mindful breathing.

Session 3 explores how and why stress and anxiety affect chest pain and offers practical ways of managing stress, including problem solving and relaxation techniques.

Session 4 explores how common, negative beliefs about activity and chest pain are unhelpful and why activity may interact with chest pain. A plan is developed to increase activity over time in a way that suits the patient's lifestyle and goals.

Session 5 focuses on how thoughts and beliefs feed the vicious cycle of chest pain. This session helps the patient find more helpful ways of thinking about chest pain.

Session 6 is a review of treatment where progress is assessed, positive changes are identified and a maintenance plan is made for the future.

The workbook is structured in this way because stress, anxiety and chest breathing are so common in NCCP. Early sessions focus on learning effective strategies such as abdominal breathing, relaxation and problem solving because they can lead to rapid improvements, which engenders confidence in the biopsychosocial approach. Patients are then better able to try more challenging interventions, such as increasing their activity and reframing their thoughts and beliefs about NCCP.

General advice for structuring sessions

In line with good CBT practice, every session begins with setting an agenda and ends with a summary and agreed-on homework tasks. Appendix 3 includes handouts to use with patients in each session, which they should take home. There is an audio guide to teach patients the breathing and relaxation skills, which can be downloaded at www.routledge.com/9781138119017. By taking weekly handouts home, patients can recap the work you have done together and better remember the session and homework tasks. Treatment success is contingent upon using the strategies regularly, requiring the patient to be motivated and able to practise and make changes at home. It is worth gently reiterating the importance of homework in every session whilst remaining aware that this can be difficult for people.

Session 1

Understanding chest pain and setting goals

Focus your questions on

- This session occurs 1–2 weeks after assessment. How has the patient's understanding of their symptoms changed as a result of the initial assessment?
- What do they expect from treatment? How might CBT apply to their chest pain?
- How do their goals for treatment link with their values in life?

Summary of session 1

1. Open the session. Welcome the patient (introduce yourself if necessary), and set the agenda for today. This session should be 1–2 weeks after the initial assessment.
2. Review the individual's chest pain cycle. Look at the physical, lifestyle, social, cognitive, behavioural and emotional factors, and find out what the patient thinks about these now that they have had time for consideration.
3. Explain that persistent chest pain in the absence of heart disease is common and benign. Give information about other, non-cardiac causes of chest pain.
4. Explain why a CBT approach can help.
5. Set boundaries for treatment (timings, number of sessions and focus) and review the session-by-session focus.
6. Set values-based SMART (specific, measurable, achievable, realistic and time-limited) goals. What does the person hope to get from therapy, and why?
7. Reassess frequency and severity of chest pain and resulting distress, in case it has changed since the initial assessment.
8. Set homework.

What you will need

- Agenda for today
- Individual's chest pain cycle completed with information from assessment (two copies: one for your notes and one for the patient)
- Copy of blank outcome measures (Appendix 2) to measure chest pain frequency, severity and interference, anxiety and depression
- Handouts 2–4 (goals for treatment, homework following session 1, chest pain diary)

Aims of session 1

This session is your opportunity to engage the patient in a collaborative therapeutic relationship. We ask where the patient would like to see themselves in the future (at 3 months, 6 months and a year) and how this is different from how they see themselves now. To be meaningful, the guided self-help should be based upon what is most important in the patient's life (their values).

Goals and values

Goals and values have motivational properties. Goals refer to specific changes and achievements that can be measured and can help to focus therapy and quantify success. Values are the foundation of meaningful goals because they identify what is really important to someone, what they wish to stand for and what gives their life meaning. A value is not achieved; it is an ongoing process – the way we live our life. Values guide decisions in what changes to make and what goals to work towards. If specific goals are linked to broader values, then therapeutic outcomes may be improved (e.g. Chase et al., 2013). This approach is central to a therapeutic method known as acceptance and commitment therapy (ACT) (e.g. Hayes and Strosahl, 2004).

The chronicity of NCCP often results in major life changes. Many people find that chest pain prevents them from living life as they used to. A therapeutic alliance is developed if the therapist can be warm, understanding and empathetic. This requires the therapist to spend time on developing a proper understanding the patient's experiences of chest pain and how these interfere with their values. The therapeutic alliance has a significant influence on therapeutic outcome, so it is worth taking time to build a collaborative working relationship based on the wish to move towards meaningful goals.

Most patients will have the goal of reducing pain. However, this goal may not always be possible and doesn't account for wider values. It is useful to ask people what they would be *doing differently* if they were pain free, and why. Regardless of pain, find out what other changes would be meaningful in the person's life. This will take time, and the biomedical view of chest pain and longing for a cure may be held tightly. Early goal-setting requires sensitive exploration of what else might be possible.

CBT is collaborative, based on guided discovery. The therapist's role includes some psychoeducation and skills-teaching, but only after the patient has expressed their point of view. People learn more effectively when they discover new information themselves and have time to reflect, test out new ideas and ask questions. The biopsychosocial approach will be novel to most people, and they will need time to test it out. A great deal of this work is done between sessions, and not all of it will eradicate chest pain, although the work can still move the patient closer to other valued goals.

CBT for NCCP is based on scientific evidence that it is effective, but everyone is different. We recommend that you present the ideas and skills in this workbook as *suggestions* to be experimented with. The chest pain cycle is a *hypothesis,* and you will work together to gather evidence about whether it is true for the patient.

Before you begin

Review the information gained from assessment and check that a chest pain cycle has been completed. If not, write the identified biological causes/physical sensations, thoughts, emotions, behaviours, social factors and protective factors in the relevant boxes. A completed example is shown in Figure 7.2. The chest pain cycle is your road map for treatment, and it can be revised each week as more information comes to light. We always ensure that both the clinician and the patient keep a copy.

Opening the first session

Welcome the patient. If you did not conduct the assessment, introduce yourself and discuss your role in guiding the treatment over the coming weeks. You could ask how they feel about seeing you and if they have expectations about what will happen. Time is limited, so you may wish to keep this brief, noting down important points to revisit in the session after you have set the agenda.

All sessions begin with setting a written agenda that identifies the main items you both wish to cover. This sets boundaries, preserves focus and supports collaboration. Good time-keeping is an important way of helping people to feel contained and safe, so inform your patient of how long the session will last, and keep to it.

You may wish to explain how treatment consists of working through a number of sessions together. These sessions have been found to benefit people with chest pain, and each one follows a specific agenda. However, there is flexibility, and you will do your best to cover any additional questions or issues by adding these to the agenda at the start of each session.

Session 1 will recap the most important points from assessment so you both start with a shared understanding of what factors might be important in their chest pain. This will be followed by an overview of treatment and setting values-based goals. Finally, there is some suggested homework. Add any other issues the patient wants to the agenda. Finally, you may wish to complete the questionnaires again to see if assessment has led to any change.

BOX W1.1 AGENDA FOR SESSION 1

Review the chest pain cycle and why thoughts, emotions, behaviours and the social world matter.
Explain chest pain.
Explain what treatment involves and how it can help.
Set values-based goals for treatment.
Provide homework.
Measure chest pain (repeat measures used in assessment).
Add additional issues to the agenda.

Reviewing the assessment and chest pain cycle

With the individual's chest pain cycle in hand, you can find out how the patient felt about the assessment, the biopsychosocial approach and the information leaflet they took home. How do they feel about this approach to chest pain? Try to use the patient's own words and phrases.

Box W1.2 gives a sample dialogue for reviewing the chest pain cycle (based on the Suzie case study in Chapter 7). As changes occur after assessment, we usually check to see if the patient has made further observations about their chest pain. The chest pain cycle is a *hypothesis*, not a definitive explanation. Treatment can be seen as an opportunity to test the hypothesis by finding out whether chest pain is improved if factors within the chest pain cycle are successfully targeted. It is always important to acknowledge scepticism and reservations; these are normal and showing your respect for this will enhance the therapeutic alliance.

BOX W1.2 SAMPLE DIALOGUE FOR REVIEWING THE CHEST PAIN CYCLE (BASED ON SUZIE IN CHAPTER 7)

Body/physical sensations: You told us how you've been having chest pain for a few months. It feels sharp, "like a dagger through the heart", and very unpleasant. You often feel breathless and faint at the same time, is that right? The doctors have done several tests and found that your heart is healthy and normal. You found this confusing because the pain really feels as if it is coming from your heart. What did the doctor think is the cause of your pain? That's right, they noted that your back injury is still causing pain, and this radiates into the chest. This is actually very common, and although it is painful, it is not dangerous. Physiotherapy might help. The muscle pain is made worse by tension and overbreathing.

Thinking and beliefs: Before you came here, you told us that nobody had explained your chest pain. Understandably, you therefore worried that something important had been missed. You read up about chest pain on the Internet, which worried you more, so you asked other doctors for help and had more tests, all with the same outcome. Now, when you get chest pain, you think it might be a heart attack or that something bad will happen. Is that right? How does this make you feel?

Emotions: Understandably, this makes you feel very scared and worried about chest pain. You think it is dangerous, so you feel anxious. As you have had chest pain for months, you now feel sad, too, because it has changed your life so much.

Behaviour: Because you haven't been offered help so far, you have to find your own ways of managing chest pain. Because you are concerned about your heart, you worry that activity could be dangerous. You also note that you get chest pain more when you're breathless. So you've stopped doing activities such as walking and seeing friends. This makes you feel sad and worried, which affects your body. When we are less active, it takes longer for injuries to heal and we lose fitness so we are likely to become breathless.

Quality of life: After your first episode of chest pain, you went to hospital and had invasive tests. This led you and your family to believe that the pain must be serious, increasing your anxiety. You are also under a lot of stress at work, and you are worried about redundancy, so you generally feel quite anxious.

Positive and protective factors: You have a very supportive family who will help you to make any changes you need. You already recognize the impact of stress on chest pain, which is a very important first step in this treatment.

Summary: Chest pain has had a profound effect on your life, and you have not had much help with it yet. Your heart is healthy, so there are other explanations. The 'vicious cycle' here can explain what is happening, and treatment here can help.

Education about NCCP and your treatment

Acknowledge scepticism

Some people with NCCP will feel immediately reassured by your explanation and recognize the CBT model as consistent with their experience. Yet many more will have some doubt about this new perspective. This is to be encouraged! Treatment is designed to test out whether the alternative explanation is correct, make room for scepticism; like a scientist you are both attempting to discover whether a new hypothesis stands up to experiments designed to test it out.

Review the facts about NCCP and normalize

By this point, all patients will have read the information leaflet after assessment (handout 1). You may like to review the facts about NCCP, how common it is and how it is not medically serious, and then discuss what the patient thinks.

Explaining why CBT is being offered

This approach offers hope to people who may not yet have received any helpful input from health-care services. We tell our patients that there is good evidence for CBT for NCCP, for example, in a recent Cochrane Review (Kisely et al., 2012). This is not because NCCP is psychological, but rather because CBT is an excellent way of giving people tools to manage (and even reduce) chest pain and giving them more control. CBT is not a cure, although many people find that it leads to important reductions in pain severity and frequency, as well as improvements in anxiety, mood and functioning.

Explaining what CBT involves

An overview of treatment helps people understand what CBT involves. It is usually a six-session format (five more after today). However, many patients find that they don't need all of these sessions, particularly if changes are seen quickly, and you both feel this would be best. Box W1.3 is an example of how you might explain the treatment to a patient.

BOX W1.3 SAMPLE DIALOGUE FOR EXPLAINING NCCP AND THE GUIDED SELF-HELP TREATMENT

Recurrent chest pain in the absence of any heart problems is extremely common. It affects 30% of people in the UK, Europe and the US. Specialist chest pain clinics report that three quarters of their patients have pain that is *unrelated* to their heart. These other possible causes of chest pain have good medical prognoses. Most chest pain clinics are set up to manage cardiac-related risk, which means they only test for and rule out heart disease. These clinics do not try to identify alternative causes for the pain, so they are unlikely to provide the appropriate help, and chest pain can become persistent.

The most common medical causes of chest pain are: **pain from muscles between the ribs** (from tension in these muscles), **pain in the chest wall** (from strains in the muscles or ligaments) and from **unhelpful breathing** (breathing too fast and using the chest muscles), **digestive causes** (acid reflux or spasm in the food pipe or ulcers) or **pain from pinched nerves** in the neck or back, which radiates and feels as if it is in the chest. Sometimes there is no underlying medical problem that can be identified, and sometimes chest pain is caused by **stress or anxiety**. None of these are medically serious and are usually treatable. If not treated pain persists, possibly for a long time.

Persistence of chest pain without treatment understandably leads people to worry about what is happening. They often think there is something seriously wrong. This way of thinking affects how they feel and what they do.

Why treatment with CBT

Some people will find that their pain significantly improves simply by having the cause identified and treated. Other people need a bit more support with changing some of the other factors in their chest pain cycle. This is where CBT can help. CBT is a psychological therapy, but this does not mean that your pain is not real. It means that you can learn self-management skills to help you cope with chest pain, to reduce your worry and distress and to improve your quality of life and general well-being. Research has found that CBT sometimes makes chest pain less severe and less frequent. It may not be a complete cure, and chest pain may still continue. However, you may notice other enhancements in your well-being, depending on the specific factors that are affecting your chest pain.

Setting values-based goals

Goals sometimes emerge in assessment. Detailed investigation will identify what is important to the patient, other than becoming 'chest pain free'. Bear in mind the need to connect with the individual's *values*. This may require a dialogue about what is most important in the patient's life, what they stand for, and how chest pain inhibits this. Sometimes you may need to point to possible domains of values, such as health, relationships (family, friends, intimate), community, hobbies, work, spirituality and so on.

Use what you already know to help, as you have probably discussed the impact of chest pain on someone's life and, in particular, how chest pain interfered with an ability to engage with aspects of life that are particularly important or meaningful. You could ask what being chest pain free would lead to – what would the person do, think or feel if this happened. Alternatively, explore what might improve their life even if chest pain continues.

When you have identified what values are important to the individual, you can use these to set more precise goals using the SMART goal approach:

- Specific
- Measurable

- Achievable
- Realistic
- Time-limited

Some questions you may wish to use to help elicit values and set related SMART goals are suggested in Box W1.4. Ideally you will have more than one goal (probably three or four) that have associated behavioural or cognitive changes.

BOX W1.4 QUESTIONS TO HELP YOU WITH GOAL-SETTING

You may find it helpful to use some of the following questions (you probably won't need them all):

- What do you hope to get out of having treatment here?
- Apart from reducing chest pain, what are your top three goals for treatment?
- What do you value most in your life? (You can give examples here, such as family, friends, work, community, religion or spirituality.)
- If chest pain was less of a problem, what would be different in your life or what would you be *doing* differently?
- Has chest pain affected or prevented you from doing things that you value in your life? What things, and how?
- If you are still doing some things you value at the moment, despite chest pain, how would you like to build on these?

Specific: Can we make these specific?
Measureable: How could we measure these goals so we can both see whether things are changing?
Achievable: How confident do you feel in being able to achieve these goals? Can you rate this from 0–10? What would make you feel more confident?
Realistic: Is this how you were living your life before chest pain began?
Time-limited: This goal (for example, getting back to full-time work/running the London marathon) is really important to you, but I wonder if it may take you longer achieve than the 6 weeks we have to work together. What shorter and mid-term goals would you need to reach first to help you on the way to achieving these longer-term goals (e.g. doing 2 days a week at work/running for 20 minutes 3 times a week)?

For example, Suzie's initial goals were to have less chest pain and worry less about it. When exploring her values, Suzie identified that family life, good friendships, working and feeling better about herself were very important and that chest pain had affected all of these. We developed the following SMART goals that were in line with her values:

Family

- To return to cooking for the family, beginning with one meal a week and working up to three meals a week
- To spend more time with the kids; to take teenage daughter shopping and to watch son's football team

Friends

- To meet a friend for coffee in town once every fortnight
- To go swimming with a friend each week like I used to

Work

- To return to the same number of hours at work as I did before (20 hours per week)

Self-care

- To learn how to manage stress more effectively and keep active by walking to places like I used to

These specific goals reflected what was important to Suzie whilst also being measurable and largely achievable within the time frame of therapy. They gave us a clear focus for treatment.

Measuring chest pain

Standardized outcome measures help you both measure change, and we suggest at least using measures of chest pain. However, as this may not change for everyone, you may like to measure levels of depression, anxiety, activity and functioning as well. These are discussed in Chapter 7 and available in Appendix 2. In our clinic we repeat these measures at the start of every session as a way of monitoring change. You may like to do this, perhaps by including them as part of homework task.

Homework following session 1

Session 1 is your opportunity to set a precedent for homework (activities such as reading therapy notes, thinking about your discussions, practicing new skills and keeping a diary). We really emphasize the benefits of homework whilst acknowledging that it is normal for people to struggle to find time, space and energy to do it. You can preempt potential problems with homework by asking how the patient thinks they will manage homework and what will make it easier for them. You can reflect on their goals and values to help them see the importance of prioritizing treatment, including work done at home. Sometimes it helps to point out that treatment is only for a few weeks and then ask if commitment to homework tasks over this limited time period is possible.

Homework for session 1 is an opportunity for the patient to read through the paperwork done in therapy and think about your discussions. They can take home a copy of their chest pain cycle, goals, treatment plan and clinic information to read. You can encourage them to note down any questions that arise over the week or to add to the chest pain cycle or goals if new ideas come to them.

We find it useful to ask the patient to keep a chest pain diary where they can identify common triggers that may not yet have been noticed. The homework list for session 1 and the chest pain diary are available in handouts 3 and 4. You can demonstrate what to write by going through the example in the first row of the diary.

Homework

- Take home the clinic information leaflet and your chest pain cycle. Think about what we have discussed today and whether this might apply to your own experience of chest pain.
- Take home a copy of your goals, and add in any new goals if they arise.
- Keep a chest pain diary over the next week. Note down chest pain whenever it happens, and try to include triggers (what happened before) and reactions, including anything that seems to help.

References

Chase, J.A., Houmanfar, R., Hayes, S.C., Ward, T.A., Vilardaga, J.P., & Follette, V. (2013). Values are not just goals: Online ACT-based values training adds to goal setting in improving undergraduate college student performance. *J Context Behav Sci* 2(3–4): 79–84.

Hayes, S.C., & Strosahl, K.D. (2004). *A practical guide to acceptance and commitment therapy*. New York: Springer-Verlag.

Kisely, S.R., Campbell, L.A., Yelland, M.J., & Paydar, A. (2012). Psychological interventions for symptomatic management of non-specific chest pain in patients with normal coronary anatomy (Review). *Cochrane Database Syst Rev* 6: CD004101.

Rimes, K.A., Wingrove, J., Moss-Morris, R., & Chalder, T. (2014). Competencies required for the delivery of high and low-intensity cognitive behavioural interventions for Chronic Fatigue, Chronic Fatigue Syndrome/ME and Irritable Bowel Syndrome. *Behav Cogn Psychother* 42(6): 760–4.

Session 2

Paced, mindful, abdominal breathing

Focus your questions on

- What is the patient's understanding of chest pain since the last session?
- Can the patient understand the role of chest versus abdominal breathing in chest pain?
- Is the person able to practise abdominal breathing at home and assess how it affects chest pain and stress levels?

Summary of session 2

1. Open the session with agenda setting, review of homework and bridge to last session regarding the chest pain cycle.
2. Provide education about chest breathing and its relationship to physiological (muscular strain) and psychological factors (stress and anxiety) in chest pain.
3. Provide education about, demonstration of and teaching of abdominal breathing. Mention link to mindfulness techniques.
4. Explain and test out how abdominal breathing can be used to manage chest pain by reducing physiological and (if relevant) psychological issues that trigger or result from chest pain.
5. Set homework.

What you will need

- Written agenda for session 2
- Copy of individual's chest pain cycle and goals
- Script for guided breathing exercise
- A pillow/mat/bed if patient wishes to lie down (optional)
- Handouts 5 and 6 (helpful breathing and homework following session 2)
- Audio CD or access to the audio guide for breathing exercises
- Coloured dot stickers (optional)

Aims of session 2

This session is the first opportunity to test out a practical strategy to help with chest pain. It is a chance to find out if changing one specific part of the chest pain cycle (breathing) effects chest pain. The breathing technique is paced, mindful abdominal breathing (also referred to as *diaphragmatic breathing*). It benefits most patients, even if overbreathing was not identified in assessment. Abdominal breathing can have broad physiological and emotional effects: it reduces chest strain, anxiety and stress, and it helps divert attention away from worry. It offers a practical skill which can help the patient feel more in control. Patients in our clinic have described abdominal breathing as the most useful specific skill they learn in therapy. In many cases, it led to a significant and fast improvement in their chest pain symptoms. Some of their comments about this are shown in Box W2.1.

BOX W2.1 COMMENTS FROM PATIENTS ABOUT PACED ABDOMINAL BREATHING

"The breathing reduced my chest pain so fast, in the first two weeks of coming here. I'm using it a lot of the time still."

"Abdominal breathing made my chest pain better. I do it a lot . . . it is easier to do the breathing now, even if the chest pain is bad."

"Now if I feel stress, I use breathing which helps hugely."

"It helps me just to focus on my breathing."

"The abdominal breathing has become natural now."

"My chest pain reduced initially with the breathing, my children are happier because I am happier, so I want to keep this up."

"I'm breathing all the time."

The ability to manage or control chest pain independently is a novel and powerful experience for most patients. If breathing strategies are effective, they provide compelling evidence in support of the biopsychosocial chest pain cycle. If chest pain can be improved through a very simple change in breathing, then assumptions about the cause of chest pain are challenged. Patients often being to realize that chest pain cannot be cardiac in origin, so the alternative explanation may be valid instead.

Most of our NCCP patients have a tendency to use chest breathing, regardless of other factors in their chest pain cycle. Some do have respiratory disorders or hyperventilation syndrome, anxiety or panic, but even if such issues are not present, abdominal breathing is still helpful. Chest breathing may not be the most significant cause of chest pain, but it often exacerbates it. We refer to previous findings that breath-holding induced pain in approximately 40% of our patients. Chest breathing can put strain on the chest wall and intercostal muscles, so changing breathing patterns can rapidly reduce strain. We use this physiological explanation with all patients because it makes intuitive sense. Breathing also impacts autonomic (stress) arousal. Depending on the factors relevant to your patient, additional explanation around paced breathing and stress management may also be useful. Ideally, present the relevance of abdominal breathing so that it fits with the individual's chest pain cycle. Try to take into account whether a patient prefers physiological or psychological explanations, and if they have not acknowledged the importance of stress, you may prefer to keep a physiological focus.

Opening session 2

Begin by welcoming the patient and briefly ask how they have been since their last session. Set today's agenda (Box W2.2) and ensure you note down anything else the patient would like to address.

BOX W2.2 AGENDA FOR SESSION 2

Review homework: identify triggers and responses to chest pain and update the chest pain cycle.
Understand how we breathe and how chest breathing affects pain.
Understand how paced, abdominal, mindful breathing can help.
Learn to use paced, abdominal, mindful breathing.
Set homework.
Address any additional issues.

Homework review

It is good practice to begin with a bridge to the previous session by checking for patient's thoughts about what was discussed and how they have managed over the last week. Explore any developments in their understanding of chest pain, and check if there is anything they don't understand or are unhappy with. Remember that being open to the patient's experience is central to building a collaborative relationship and therapeutic alliance. It usually takes 5 to 10 minutes to open the session and review homework.

As homework is central to treatment success, demonstrate its importance every session by looking through their diary and asking about what they have noticed. If the diary was not completed, it is still important to ask about chest pain and link back to the patient's chest pain cycle Note any new information that arises.

1 When did the chest pain happen? Are there usual times, places, people, activities or behaviours associated with it?
2 How did you usually feel (emotionally) when you have chest pain?

3 What thoughts did you have about chest pain? Is there a theme?
4 What did you do in reaction to chest pain?
5 What did other people do in reaction to chest pain?
6 How long did the chest pain episodes last? Did anything stop them?
7 What happened when the chest pain stopped?
8 Did you notice how these things affected each other? Did you notice any patterns?
9 How does this fit with your chest pain cycle?

Understanding how we breathe

Explain that today you would like to teach a new skill that may help them to respond to chest pain more effectively and to feel more in control. You may like to mention the evidence for this skill. We usually begin with a physiological rationale for abdominal breathing, which is as a technique that reduces strain around the chest wall. For patients who are already aware and open to the concept of stress affecting chest pain, you may like to explain how breathing exercises are an effective stress management tool. This is less advisable for people who do not acknowledge the role of stress. Try to maintain the spirit of collaboration and guided discovery; remember that you are offering a new skill that has worked for other people, but you can only discover if it will help them by experimenting with it.

The overbreathing test

This will probably have been covered in assessment, but it can be useful to repeat it in treatment. It offers a powerful demonstration of how chest breathing can trigger pain. Follow the instructions in Box W2.3.

BOX W2.3 HOW TO DO THE OVERBREATHING TEST

Give your patient the following instructions. It is supportive if you do the test together, both overbreathing at the same time.

"For the next 30 seconds I would like us to see what happens when we breathe quickly, using our chest muscles. What do you predict will happen?"

You can note down their predictions and then begin overbreathing together. If you can't see their chest moving, ask them to try taking deeper breaths. After about 30 seconds, stop the test. Ask them how they are feeling. Specifically ask about how they are feeling physically (e.g. chest pain or discomfort, tension, dizzy, light-headed) or emotionally (e.g. more anxious or stressed).

Most people will feel something. Compare this to their predictions and ask what they think this means.

The overbreathing test can show the power breathing styles have on the body. Overbreathing may lead to chest pain, in which case you can refer to the chest pain cycle, emphasizing how chest pain and strain of the chest wall are related. This is a nonthreatening cause of chest pain. Overbreathing may not cause pain, in which case, compare how the patient feels after overbreathing to how they feel when they begin to use abdominal breathing, next on the agenda.

Abdominal breathing

You may like to use handout 5 to support you. We usually begin with an explanation of why abdominal breathing is relevant to chest pain (Box W2.4).

BOX W2.4 SAMPLE EXPLANATION ABOUT HOW CHEST BREATHING AFFECTS CHEST PAIN

Breathing depends on us drawing air into the lungs. The lungs are in a cavity in the chest. They do not have any muscle around them, so in order to draw air into the lungs, our body has to expand the cavity surrounding the lungs. This can be done using the chest or using the diaphragm. The chest is expanded when we use the muscles around the chest and shoulders to lift the ribs up and out. This is called *chest breathing.* The diaphragm is a dome-shaped muscle below the lungs which can expand the lungs downwards if we flatten it. This is *abdominal breathing,* because when the diaphragm moves down, our abdomen expands.

When you did the overbreathing test, you were breathing in the way that most people breathe if they are doing strenuous activity or feeling excited or stressed. This is normal but can cause some difficulties if we breathe in this way all of the time, because chest breathing can cause discomfort and pain.

Think about what happens when we use the chest to breathe. What did you notice moving? That's right . . . the chest and shoulders move up and down, expanding so that air is drawn into the lungs. The breath is fast, irregular, shallow or gasping. Since the muscles around your chest and rib cage are working hard to move, they get tired and can be strained. Often this muscle strain causes pain, and it is commonly this that leads to chest pain. People who tend to rely on their chest to breathe may be more likely to strain these muscles and have chest pain. This type of breathing can also cause other sensations, such as breathlessness; struggling to breathe; finding breathing exhausting; feeling restricted, trapped or confined; dizziness, headache, blurred vision, muscle tension in the chest and elsewhere; and palpitations. None of these are dangerous, but they can feel very unpleasant.

Check for understanding and answer any questions. You can then move on to describing and demonstrating abdominal breathing, possibly using the sample explanations in Boxes W2.5 and W2.6. We also find it helps to show patients a diagram of abdominal breathing (Figure W2.1), which is also available in handout 5.

BOX W2.5 EXAMPLE SCRIPT OF HOW TO TEACH ABDOMINAL BREATHING

A more helpful way of breathing will reduce tension around the chest wall by using the diaphragm instead. Remember that in order to breathe, all we need to do is expand the cavity around the lungs. The diaphragm is an alternative means to expand the lungs. The diaphragm is a dome-shaped muscle at the bottom of the lungs. [Point at the diagram of abdominal breathing.]

To take a breath in, we contract the diaphragm and it becomes flat. The lungs expand into this space, and air is drawn in. The diaphragm is a very efficient muscle and, unlike the chest wall muscles, it does not become fatigued or strained. As the diaphragm flattens, it will push down slightly on the organs in the stomach, so the stomach itself will push outwards. So when we use abdominal breathing, the abdomen will expand as we breathe in and fall flat when we breathe out. This movement of the abdomen is why we call it abdominal breathing.

Abdominal breathing is natural. If you look at people sleeping, or if you see how children and babies breathe, you will notice how their abdomen moves with the breath, rather than their chest. We all start out using abdominal breathing, but then we can get into bad habits perhaps because of environmental changes such as chronic stress or bad posture, weight gain or tight clothing. The good news is that we can learn to reverse this habit and return to using abdominal breathing more often.

Demonstration in the session

It is easiest to teach abdominal breathing if you can give a live demonstration. With the patient watching, place one of your hands on your chest and the other on your abdomen. Begin by showing chest

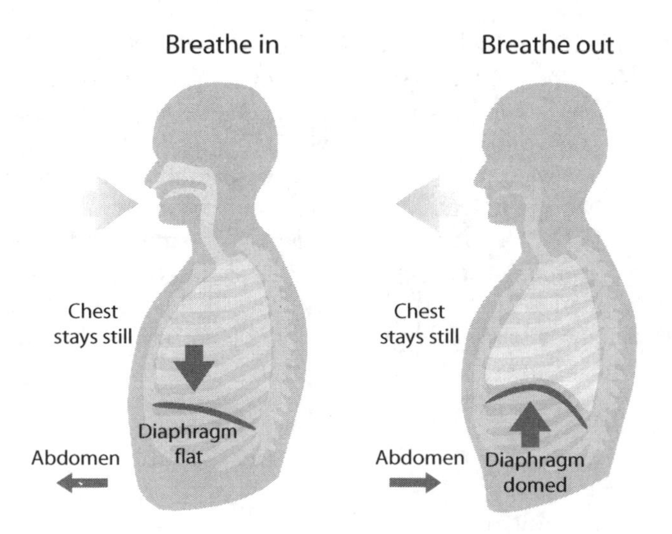

Figure W2.1 Diagram demonstrating abdominal breathing styles

breathing and take a few deep chest breaths, pointing out how the chest moves whilst the abdomen is still. Next, change to taking a few abdominal breaths, pointing out how the chest is now still whilst the abdomen moves up and down. You may wish to exaggerate the breathing to show the movement, noting how the abdomen expands as you breathe in and deflates as you breathe out.

The patient can then try for themselves. Ask them to place their hands in the same positions on their body. First they can try a normal breath, and if the chest moves, this is a sign of chest breathing. Next the patient can try abdominal breathing. Encourage them to do this slowly and not too deeply. It is easier to do lying down, but if this is not possible, they could stand up, as this creates more room for the diaphragm to move. Further guidance is given in Box W2.6.

BOX W2.6 HOW TO TEACH ABDOMINAL BREATHING

It can take a while to learn abdominal breathing, so be gentle with yourself and just see what happens. With one hand on your chest and the other on your abdomen, take in a breath slowly, but not too deeply. Try to keep the chest still. Imagine that the breath is travelling all the way down the body into the stomach area. As you breathe in, the diaphragm contracts, pushing your abdomen outwards. It can help you to imagine that the breath travels to your stomach, filling it with air so it expands.

Now breathe out slowly, allowing the air to flow back up the body and out of your mouth or nose (it doesn't matter which). As you breathe out your diaphragm relaxes back to its domed shape. This means the abdomen returns to its relaxed, flatter position. Again, it might help to imagine that you are breathing out of your stomach and the air is being pushed out of the abdomen. All the while the chest stays still.

Keep breathing slowly and steadily. You can try counting: breathe in, 1, 2, 3, let the breath turn around and breathe out, 1, 2, 3, and allow there to be a slight space before taking the next breath in. Don't breathe too deeply, or you may feel a bit dizzy. If you start to feel light-headed, then breathe less deeply and slow it down. Your stomach muscles should be relaxed so they move with the breath, rising as you breathe in and flattening as you breathe out.

Aim for about 8 to 12 smooth, steady breaths a minute. Try to resist gasping, throat clearing or coughing.

Some people learn this skill easily, some require a lot of practise and a small minority struggle to develop the skill fully. Reassure anyone struggling that it is normal to need practise. In learning this new skill, they have to change the habit of a lifetime. Encourage them to be kind to themselves and to give themselves plenty of time to practise at home using the audio guide and handouts.

Short guided breathing exercise

Ideally you will have at least 5 minutes to guide the patient in a breathing exercise, with the patient lying down, if this is not possible then ask them to stand (to allow the diaphragm maximum expansion). This exercise is an opportunity to model a slow and gentle breathing style regardless of what else might be happening in the moment. If they report a racing mind or discomfort in the body, encourage them to learn how to keep gently keep refocusing their attention back onto the breath in the abdomen whenever it wanders off. The breathing exercise provided here is based on some principles of mindfulness (see Box W2.7 for a word on mindfulness). The advantage of this approach is that, even if a patient cannot master the abdominal technique, they can still benefit from learning how to pace their breath, how to use the breath as a focus for attention and how to be aware of sensations in the body without having to judge or change them.

Box W2.8 gives a sample script for the guided breathing exercise. It is similar to the audio guide the patient will take home, but you may find that you only have a few minutes to do this in the session, so it is shorter. Afterwards, you can ask the patient for feedback, what they noticed during the practice, how they feel now and how this compares to how they felt after overbreathing earlier in the session.

BOX W2.7 A WORD ON MINDFULNESS AND BREATHING

Research has found that mindfulness practice can lead to significant improvements in the management of pain and other difficult physical symptoms (Brown and Jones, 2013) and to significant benefits in well-being (Grossman et al., 2004).

Central to mindfulness is the idea that is possible to pay attention to experiences (including difficult or painful experiences) in a way that is purposeful and nonjudgemental. This form of attention seems to lead to the development of a more compassionate and accepting attitude that is thought to be associated with significant benefits for the individual. The exercises here include some suggestions about how people can begin to gently notice and explore physical sensations without judging them or trying too hard to change them. Rather than attempting to push away or stop difficult thoughts and feelings, it is possible to learn to simply notice what is happening and then to choose to refocus attention onto the breath.

We have included this because we found that some patients are unable to learn abdominal breathing, yet they can still derive significant benefit from focusing on their breath. They can also learn how to pay attention to their body in a gentle way and to use the breath as a place to focus their attention on something rhythmic at times of stress and pain. This type of exercise typically leads to an automatic slowing down of the breath, which will lead to a sense of calmness and a reduction of the physiological correlates of anxiety.

The topic of mindfulness is large and complex and outside the scope of this book. For further resources, see Section 3.

BOX W2.8 SCRIPT FOR A GUIDED BREATHING EXERCISE

Try to speak slowly, pausing for several seconds (indicated in the text with ellipses).

In this exercise you are just becoming more aware of your breath and body, however they feel now . . . Not having to judge or change anything, but simply paying attention to your body and scanning through it. Beginning with your feet, notice what you feel here . . . moving up to your ankles, lower legs . . . knees and upper legs . . . . No need to change anything. As best as you can, just noticing what is already here . . . Focusing on your hips and pelvic area . . . moving up to the back, feeling the length of your spine and your neck . . . feeling your arms . . . feeling your head and face . . . .

Now move attention to your chest and abdominal area . . . Can you become aware of what sensations are present in the chest? Remember, you don't have to judge or change these sensations even if they feel uncomfortable, can you just let them be . . . ? Can you just notice how they change, moment by moment . . . ?

And now focusing on your breath. If it is comfortable to do so, breathe with your diaphragm so that your chest is still and your abdomen is moving up and down. No need to breathe deeply, just slowly and steadily . . . Feel the abdomen rise as you breathe in and flatten as you breathe out . . . . The abdomen rises as you breathe in . . . falls flat at you breathe out . . . .

If you can't get the hang of this abdominal breathing, that's okay. Instead, simply focus on how the breath feels right now. You may like to focus on how the breath feels in the nostrils or throat – feeling cooler as you breathe in and warmer as you breathe out. No need to struggle or fight with the breath, just allow your attention to rest on the breath moment by moment.

You will probably notice that sometimes your mind wanders away from the breath, and instead of feeling the breath you find yourself thinking about something else . . . perhaps you are thinking about what is happening in the body . . . perhaps you feel bored or sleepy or distracted . . . This is normal, and not a problem at all. The mind will keep wandering in this way. When you notice that the mind has wandered, just notice what is on your mind and then, when you are ready, you can bring your mind back to focus on the breath. . . . Can you feel the breath moving? Can you follow it all the way in and all the way out?

Just notice whatever is happening and then refocus attention onto the breath . . . . Over and over again returning attention to the breath . . . . Feeling this breath coming in . . . feeling it turn around . . . feeling this breath going out . . . .

There is no need to try and change anything right now, just allow yourself to be as you already are. The mind returning to the breath again and again. Feeling the abdomen rise with the in breath and flatten with the out breath.

Remember, the breath is always with you, always here and now. Whenever you need, you can choose to focus on the breath and connect you to this present moment . . . .

And now bringing this practice to an end, slowly open your eyes and become aware of the room around you.

Homework following session 2

The patient can take home handouts 5 and 6 (helpful breathing and homework following session 2). They will also need either a CD or the ability to download the audio guide of breathing exercises (CD tracks 1, 2 and 3) at www.routledge.com/9781138119017.

Homework

- Practise abdominal breathing for 10 minutes every day, using the audio guide. Try to schedule this in a regular daily slot. Complete the breathing diary after each practice to keep track of how it affects you and your chest pain.
- Pause and breathe several times a day. This will make abdominal breathing more habitual. Remember to stop, check your breathing and take a few slow abdominal breaths several times a day. Choose a reminder. (You can give some dot stickers to place around their home, in the car or on their phone, or they could set an alarm to remind them to stop and breathe. Find out what to use and write this down on handout 6.)
- Use abdominal breathing in response to difficulty. Once you are confident in using the technique, begin to use it as a skilled way of responding to difficulty. This may be when you are faced with a stressful situation, you feel anxious or you have chest pain. Try this only when you have had a chance to practise the technique for a few days, and then see what happens. You can then record this on the breathing diary.

References

Brown, C.A., & Jones, A.K. (2013). Psychobiological correlates of improved mental health in patients with musculoskeletal pain after a mindfulness-based pain management program. *Clin J Pain* 29(3): 233–44.

Grossman, P., Niemann, L., Schmidt, S., & Walach, H. (2004). Mindfulness-based stress reduction and health benefits: A meta-analysis. *J Psychosom Res* 57(1): 35–43.

Session 3

Stress management and relaxation

Focus your questions on

- What was the effect of using abdominal breathing for homework? Did it affect chest pain? How does it link to the chest pain cycle?
- Were there any difficulties with doing homework? How can we manage these?
- How does the patient understand the impact of anxiety and stress on chest pain?
- What stressors are in the patient's life at the moment? Are there ways of reducing this?
- Can they learn to use relaxation strategies and practise them at home?

Summary of session 3

1. Open the session with agenda setting and review of homework tasks using abdominal breathing.
2. Provide psychoeducation about stress and anxiety and their effects on the body, including chest pain.
3. Provide practical ways of managing stress and anxiety using problem solving (if appropriate).
4. Demonstrate and teach relaxation exercises (progressive muscle relaxation and relaxing imagery).
5. Set homework.

What you will need

- Written agenda for session 3
- Copy of individual's chest pain cycle
- Copy of progressive muscle relaxation script (if you need this)
- A pillow/mat/bed if patient wishes to lie down (optional)
- Handouts 7–9 and audio guide for relaxation exercises.

Aims of session 3

Session 3 focuses explicitly on stress and anxiety, how these relate to NCCP and strategies for reduction and management. By now many patients will have already derived benefit from abdominal breathing, which may have built up their confidence in the biopsychosocial approach. If they begin to see the relevance of the different factors in the chest pain cycle, they may be better prepared to begin working directly on psychosocial factors affecting their chest pain.

The first key point to address today is that stress is normal. We all experience stress and this does not suggest that someone is unwell or unusual. People have multiple responsibilities and difficulties, and modern life is filled with potential sources of stress. Patients in our clinic frequently report stressors associated with work or unemployment, conflict in relationships, bereavement, caring responsibilities for children or older family members, difficulties with finance, housing issues, asylum status and comorbid physical and mental health problems. Persistent chest pain is *itself* a significant stressor. By the time a patient reaches treatment with you, they will probably have been in and out of the medical system receiving little support or advice. Most will be struggling to get on with their lives in spite of chest pain, doing the best they can, and some will probably describe numerous demands that compete for their time and energy. For many people these demands are often prioritized over their own well-being.

Many patients attending our clinic tell us that they find it useful to learn about stress, its origins and its impact on chest pain and quality of life. They find stress management skills (relaxation and problem solving) helpful. They also describe how stress management can effectively reduce chest pain triggers or help them control the pain, and this builds their trust in the chest pain cycle. Some of their comments are shown in Box W3.1.

BOX W3.1 WHAT PATIENTS SAID ABOUT RELAXATION AND STRESS MANAGEMENT

"I don't have chest pain any more. I think it's because I got rid of the stress in my life."

"I know pain comes on when I'm stressed, so I try to rush around less now."

"I get (my family) to help at home so I don't get so stressed anymore."

"Chest pain is better now; I'm using the relaxation exercises when I get it . . . . I try to relax and that makes it go."

"I know the pain is due to stress. I never think about my heart now. The doctor said it isn't from my heart, it's because of stress."

"After we did the problem solving I saw that I needed to get extra help for my mum. I've done this now and don't worry so much about her being on her own, this has really made me feel better, and I get chest pain much less often."

"Now if I feel stress, I know what it is and I use breathing which really helps."

Opening session 3

Begin by welcoming the patient and briefly ask how things have been since their last session and with how abdominal breathing is going. Set today's agenda together, including any additional issues from the patient, particularly if there were problems with homework.

BOX W3.2 AGENDA FOR SESSION 3

Review homework: abdominal breathing, breathing diary and updating the chest pain cycle.
Troubleshoot any problems with homework.
Understand how stress and anxiety affect chest pain.
Identify current stressors and find practical ways to minimize them.
Discuss exercises to reduce stress (progressive muscular relaxation and relaxing imagery).
Set homework.
Address any additional issues.

Homework review

Bridge to the last session and you can find out about the patient's understanding, motivation and practice of abdominal breathing. If possible, try to elicit information using open questions, and see how it supports the chest pain cycle. You can reiterate the importance of practising, so ask to see the breathing diary the patient has kept. If this has not happened, you can still use two or three of the following questions to open a discussion about their experiences over the last week:

- How did you find last week's session? Was there anything you found particularly helpful or unhelpful?
- Did you practise the breathing exercises this week?
- When did you use them? Did you try using them in response to difficulty or chest pain? What happened? What does this suggest to you?
- Did you manage to remind yourself to pause and breathe? What happened?
- Have there been any problems in practising the breathing?
- What could we do today to make it easier for you manage doing homework tasks next week?

Problems with homework will arise and are best addressed early on. By identifying the issues that impede homework, you can offer encouragement and understanding and suggest changes that will help over the rest of treatment. As this is a guided self-help approach, the work done at home is integral to treatment. You may like to show that struggling with homework is normal by sharing experiences from other patients who have found it difficult to find time or space to practise or who forget, worry that they are not doing it right or don't believe that homework will make a difference. We found many of our patients struggled to prioritize their own needs over other demands and commonly reported seeing this as being selfish or self-indulgent. This is particularly common if someone has a caring role for other people with needs (e.g. elderly parents, children or people who are unwell).

Once barriers are identified, you and the patient can find a solution that will help them make the most out of treatment by practicing what is learnt in therapy at home. It is worth spending a few minutes discussing what will work for them, as the best solutions will come from the patient themselves. If this is difficult, you can offer examples of how other people solved similar issues. Box W3.3 gives examples of problems and solutions from our clinic.

BOX W3.3 DEALING WITH BARRIERS TO HOMEWORK

Problem: As a single mum with three children who works part time, Anne struggled to find any time to herself, and she would be so exhausted by the end of the day that she fell asleep whenever she tried to do the breathing exercises.

Solution: Anne decided to set her alarm 10 minutes earlier and do the exercises with her headphones on whilst still in bed, before her kids knew she was awake.

Problem: Ismael worked at a furniture store which had recently closed down the local branch, and he was moved to another store 2 hours from home. His wife was unwell, so he could not afford to leave the job. He regularly did overtime to pay the bills, so he could not find any time to do the homework exercises. He knew that stress was making his chest pain worse, but he could not see a solution because he needed all of his wages to survive.

Solution: Ismael realized that he never took his allotted 30 minute lunch each day. On discussion, he saw that the homework was important. He decided to use the disabled toilet to lie down and practise breathing exercises for 10 minutes during the lunch break each day.

Problem: Marcos prided himself on being the rock of his extended family. He was the person everyone would ask for help, he drove his mother-in-law to hospital appointments, he did the gardening for his parents, he picked up the grandkids up from school and so on. The thought of setting aside time for himself made him feel selfish. Although he wanted to make the most of treatment, he didn't remember to do the homework.

Solution: Marcos thought his wife might help and agreed to tell her what he needed to do at home. She was really supportive, told the rest of the family to give him time and reminded Marcos to practise each day after the evening meal.

Problem: Udoka did not get the hang of abdominal breathing in the session, and it was not any easier at home. She had become more and more worried about this and found herself feeling stressed whenever she tried to practise, so she gave up.

Solution: The therapist reminded Udoka that it is just as helpful to breathe slowly and focus on how the breath feels and that she could focus on the nostrils or throat if she preferred. This was easier and just focusing attention on the breath helped her to feel calmer.

Taking care of oneself

Tackling chest pain ultimately requires the patient to begin to prioritize taking care of him- or herself. This is challenging, but it is central to being able to recognize and reduce stress effectively. If stress is an important maintenance factor in the chest pain cycle, then real change depends upon the patient making this part of treatment a priority. We sometimes find it helps to use one of the analogies in Box W3.4 to highlight the importance of setting aside time to practise exercises and to take care of oneself.

BOX W3.4 ANALOGIES ABOUT THE IMPORTANCE OF TAKING CARE OF ONESELF

People often struggle to prioritize the time they need to practise the strategies they learn in treatment. However, for real change, it is important to try to find some space to do this for yourself. Perhaps the following analogy will help to show why.

Medicine analogy

Imagine that the exercises suggested are just like taking a medicine prescribed by the doctor. If your doctor prescribed a pill that you had to take once a day that might help your chest pain, would you take it? And if the same doctor said that the medication would only work if you took it daily for 6 weeks, and had to sit still for 30 minutes after taking it, what would you do? The exercises that are suggested don't include a medication, but the principle is the same. The potential benefit is also greater than any medication available for your current experiences.

Sharpening the axe metaphor (and why prioritizing self-care is important)

A young man decided to become a wood-cutter. He applied for the job and, on the first day, he felled 10 trees with his axe. The foreman was impressed and gave the man a job. The young man worked nonstop all week chopping. On the second day, he felled an impressive eight trees, on the third day he felled five trees, on the fourth day he felled two trees and on the last day he didn't manage to fell any trees at all. The young man was disheartened as he went to the foreman to collect his payment. The foreman asked what had happened exactly, and the young man told him that he had worked nonstop all week chopping. The foreman thought for a few moments and asked, "so when did you find time to sharpen your axe?"

The point is that in order to be able to meet the demands in life and the needs of other people, we first need to take time to sharpen our own axe; we have a duty to take care of ourselves.

Physical symptoms of physiological (stress) arousal and how these relate to chest pain

You can now focus on psychoeducation about stress and the body. You may find it helps to have handout 7 for this. If the patient acknowledges stress as a relevant factor, you can simply use the explanation in Box W3.5, checking the patient's understanding throughout. For those who are less aware of stress or deny its relevance, then you can begin by framing the explanation differently. For example, you can focus on how chest pain has become a cause for concern, irritation or frustration. Alternately, the demands of a busy life (work or caring etc.) can be regarded not as stress, but more like having to lift heavy weights repeatedly. Over time, lifting heavy weights can put a strain on the body, no matter how strong someone is. In this analogy, we can see the normal demands of life as weights that can overstretch the body.

An imaginary task can bring this explanation to life. You can ask the patient to imagine that are under threat; for example, the person is walking alone late at night and footsteps rapidly come up behind them. What might they feel? What body sensations might they experience? Alternately, you could ask them to remember a recent situation when they felt worried and what this was like in their body. It is useful during your explanation, and when the patient describes their own stress reactions, to point out common effects of stress and anxiety by showing them Figure W3.1.

BOX W3.5 HOW TO DESCRIBE AND EXPLAIN STRESS AND ANXIETY

Stress and anxiety are normal reactions to threat. They cause changes in our body and mind that are designed to prepare us to cope with this threat. When faced with potential danger, the body automatically releases noradrenaline (a hormone). The hormone's effect on the body makes it ready to fight or run away from the threat. This is the *fight or flight response.* Adrenaline increases the breathing rate (and often leads to more chest breathing). It makes the heart beat faster, pumping more oxygen to the muscles. The muscles are primed for action, becoming tense. Sweating may start, preparing the body to stay cool in action. The senses (sight and hearing) sharpen. Attention focuses on the possible threat, preparing the individual for a swift response.

The fight or flight response is evolutionarily adaptive. Our ancestors were more likely to survive in dangerous environments if they could respond quickly to threat. For example, the survival of our species depended on being able to escape or defend immediately and effectively if hunting in the jungle and faced with a tiger.

In modern life, the fight or flight response is less effective because the sources of threat are often chronic and complex. They are rarely resolved by fight or flight. For example, we may have everyday worries about work, money or relationships that are not easy to change. However, the brain continues to respond to these more complex, chronic threats in the same way as it does to acute danger. We react to these complex threats in the same way, as if we were coming face to face with a tiger, and we experience the physiological changes that involves.

This is relevant to chest pain, because the fight or flight response involves real, physical changes, including changes that affect sensations in the chest. These body sensations are *not dangerous*; they are just normal reactions to stress or anxiety. However, many people worry that these sensations mean there is something is wrong.

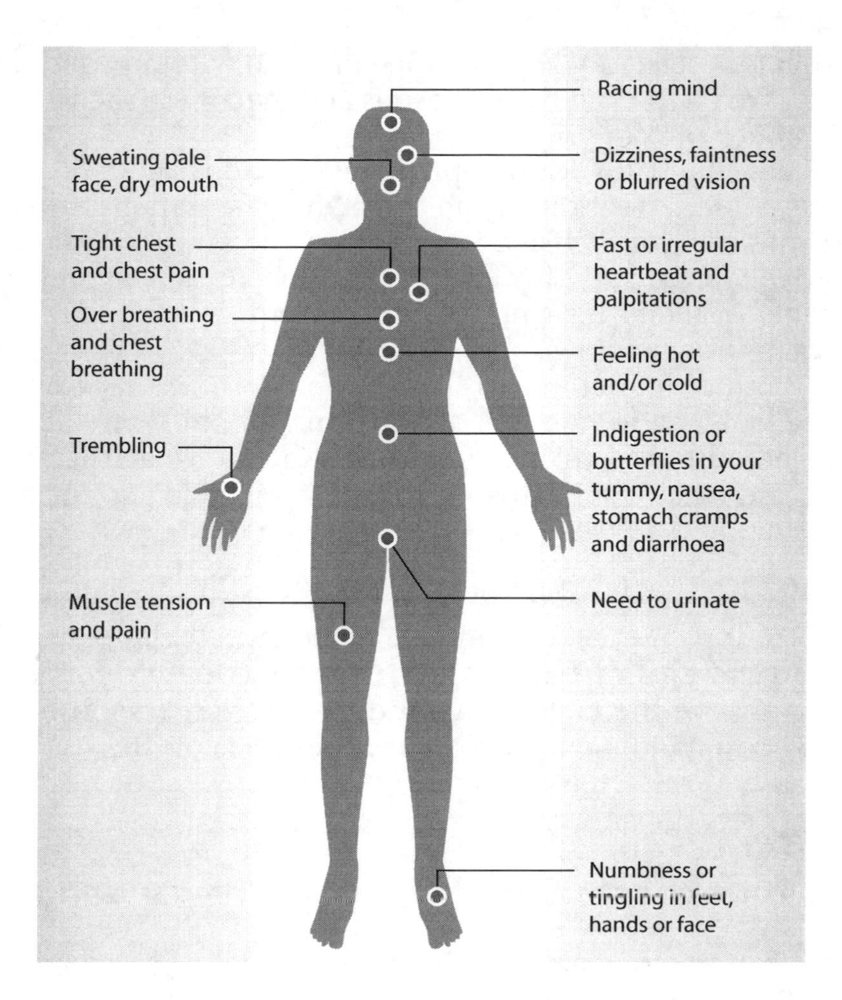

Figure W3.1 Physical sensations and physiological changes that can occur with stress

Increases in heart and breathing rates and muscle tension are common correlates of stress, and chest sensations are associated with overbreathing, tension in the chest wall and palpitations. Clearly, stress has significant implications for chest pain. We sometimes tell our patients about a survey we did with over 600 people (Marks & Hunter, unpublished manuscript). We asked people to report what happened in their bodies when they recalled a stressful past event. Chest sensations were one of the most commonly reported physical changes (reported by 53% of people), along with changes in sensations in the stomach, head and neck/shoulders. This is a really important point: chest sensations (including pain and palpitations) normally occur with stress. It does not mean there is anything seriously wrong, and they can happen even with relatively minor stress (such a remembering a past stressful event).

No matter what is causing stress and anxiety, once they have occurred, a vicious circle can easily develop in the following way:

- An event happens that causes us stress or anxiety.
- This leads to changes in our body, which might include chest sensations, pain or breathlessness.

- We don't understand what is happening and we worry about what is wrong. We focus on possible reasons and outcomes, such as having a heart attack or collapsing.
- This understandably leads to powerful emotions and more anxiety.
- We pay more attention to the threatening sensations. This narrow focus of attention is like a spotlight on the sensations, and we are sensitive to even very tiny changes in our body, which previously we probably wouldn't have notice. This confirms our worst fears and so makes us more anxious.
- We try and do something to stop the anxiety and sensations such as resting or going to hospital. This might help, but only in the short term, because we will remain worried about what the sensations mean and what would have happened if we hadn't stopped or gone to hospital.

Handout 7 describes the stress process, and you may like to use the patient's chest pain cycle to demonstrate how stress can play an important part in chest pain, even if there is nothing seriously wrong. You may like to emphasize the factors involved in the stress response by filling out the box on handout 7 ("My own vicious cycle of stress").

Identifying your stressors and practical stress management

Next, you can explore specific stressors in your patient's life. If you do not have these from assessment, then questions similar to the following may help:

- You've mentioned that sometimes you have pressure at work. Do you think this causes you any stress or anxiety? Can you tell me a bit more about what is happening at work?
- You've told me that you have a lot of responsibilities at home, with two young children and your elderly father to take care of. This sounds like it could be a possible source of stress for you. What do you think?
- Do you think that you have any sources of stress in your own life? Is there anything that you tend to worry about? Are there demands in your life that you find it difficult to keep up with?
- People with chest pain often tell me that they have things in their lives which cause them stress. This may not always be immediately obvious, but examples may include problems at work with colleagues, too big a workload, financial problems, difficulties with family or friends, bereavement or other chronic health problems. Is anything similar happening in your life?

Any new stressors can be added to the chest pain cycle. You can then use one of the following options to help target and reduce them.

Managing stress

Sometimes social factors reported by the patient may need you to refer them for specialist advice from charities or public services that offer practical support.

Examples of when referral was needed in our clinic

Mary described conflict in her marriage. Although still living with her husband, their relationship had broken down. He had refused her requests for him to leave, and instead stayed at home all day drinking. He was verbally abusive and although no longer physically abusive, he had been several years ago. Mary had no space at home to herself, and she was very unhappy. We gave her some information about sources of help:

- Information about refuges for victims of domestic violence
- Information about Alcoholics Anonymous groups for relatives of alcoholics.

She then engaged in some problem solving (see next section) and decided to make time for herself outside of the home by offering to cat-sit for her friend once a week.

Adibe was a refugee from Somalia who was seeking asylum status. He had some legal help and was waiting to hear the results of his last appeal. He was depressed and socially isolated, with no family or friends nearby. He spent most of his days alone at home, which was stressful because his neighbours were noisy and he didn't feel very safe. We gave Adibe information about:

- A local charity for the Somalian diaspora
- Attending day centre and weekly activities at the local MIND centre as a way of getting out of the house regularly.

Joanne's work was a source of stress because a colleague was bullying her. This colleague was a peer (not a superior) but kept telling Joanne what work she should do and would complain about her to other colleagues. Joanne's work was suffering and she didn't know what to do. We suggested that Joanne discuss the issues with her manager or HR team and also gave her some information about assertiveness training classes.

Problem solving

This is a practical way patients can find their own solutions, and handout 8 guides you through the process. Begin by choosing *one* practical problem causing stress that the patient wants to change. If the problem seems complicated and insurmountable, it should be broken down into smaller parts, and one part should be solved at a time. This technique can be learnt in session and then applied by the patient to other problems.

Ask the patient to think of any and all possible solutions to the problem. To encourage creativity and open-mindedness, don't judge any responses, and no matter how wacky or unlikely they are, write them down. Each possibility is considered for pros and cons, including possible consequences. The solution with the most pros and least cons is chosen. Then a plan is made to test out this solution. The plan should be specific, identifying what, when, where and how the patient will complete the plan and how they will manage any barriers. Ideally the patient will be confident to try the solution at home and to talk about the outcome in your next session. Problem solving is often an iterative process, and the initial plan may need to be modified and tried out again.

Example of problem solving

Peter was retired from working as a building site manager. He missed his job and was spending a lot of time at home, which he shared with his wife and three teenage children. Peter found the home environment stressful because his children were constantly arguing. Whenever he tried to stop the arguments, he would end up shouting at the kids. Often his wife would intervene, which made him feel undermined and upset. This often resulted in anger, breathlessness and chest pain. You can see his process of problem solving in Table W3.1.

Table W3.1 Example of Peter's problem-solving process

Identify the specific problem What do you want to achieve? Break down complex problems into smaller, easier parts.	Children arguing repeatedly at home, playing me and my wife against one another. I want to reduce their arguments, and when they do argue, I want to not be so affected by it.
Brainstorm: Write down *any* and *all* possible solutions. Have an open mind and don't judge any solutions yet.	– Send children away from home. – Move out of home. – Get wife to deal with arguments alone. – Get children to stop arguing completely. – Set some rules for the whole family about how to deal with arguments.
Consequences: Write down the pros and cons of each solution. What are the consequences of each?	– If children or I left home, this would solve the problem but break up the family. – My wife would get much more stressed which could affect our relationship negatively. – The children would struggle never to argue and might feel blamed. – Setting some rules for all of us could improve the whole family and not blame one person.
Choose the best solution: Look at pros and cons of each.	Set some rules for the whole family about how to deal with arguments.

Plan it. Make a careful plan about how to try this solution. What will you do and how will you do it? When? Where? Will anyone help you? Are there potential problems? Can you avoid them?	My wife and I will agree on the rules which usually create arguments (e.g. use of the TV and computer and setting a daily roster to be fair). *The following will be explained to the children:* Shouting is making dad feel unwell, so shouting will lead to a reduction in time on the TV or computer. If arguments are resolved calmly without shouting, there will be a reward of extra TV or computer time. The TV and computer roster is set by mum and dad and will be kept to. *If the children continue to shout after being reminded of the rules:* I will leave the room, ask my wife to deal with the kids if nearby. I will then take a walk and do breathing exercises.
Do it. Did you follow your plan?	My wife and I agreed on some extra rules, and we sat down and explained our reasons to the kids.
Evaluate it. What happened? Did you progress at all? Were there any problems with the plan?	The children were supportive when we told them about the chest pain. The arguments still happen, but they stop quickly now if I ask them calmly to stop. My eldest daughter has also begun to help by asking her brothers to keep it down when they begin to argue. I have had less chest pain as a result.
If you solved your problem, what do you need to do to keep going? If you solved just one part of a larger problem, repeat this exercise with the other parts.	The problem is mostly solved. I think we may need to revisit the rules every now and again as a family.
If your problem is not solved, how can you make a more effective plan, or can you choose an alternative solution from your list?	At the moment, the plan is quite effective, and I will continue to use it and see what happens.

Some patients will not have any particular problems that require this type of approach. If this is the case, you can move directly onto the next agenda item: applied relaxation.

Applied Relaxation

Applied relaxation targets both physiological and psychological causes of chest pain. Like breathing, it is relevant to most patients, regardless of current stress levels. Chest pain is often linked to muscle tension, particularly around the ribs, shoulders and back. Tension may be from injury, postural problems or stress. Applied relaxation exercises work by reducing muscle tension, regardless of the cause, and so it is another way to reduce causes of chest pain.

It is best to carry out the relaxation exercises with the patient in the session, so they can see what the instructions mean and ask questions. The patient can be lying down, if possible, but sitting is fine too. The first exercise (progressive muscle relaxation) works through each muscle group in the body in turn, tensing and then relaxing it. This helps people to recognize how tension feels and then how to let tension go. The second exercise (imagery) relaxes the mind, using imagination to think of a place that helps them to feel calm and relaxed.

Before you begin, ask the patient to use a scale of 0 to 10 (where 0 = none and 10 = worst imaginable) to rate current levels of

- stress,
- tension and
- any chest pain.

You can teach relaxation using the script provided in Box W3.6, which takes approximately 10 minutes. Afterwards, ask the patient to rate their levels of stress, tension and chest pain and compare these to the earlier ratings. You can emphasize any changes that might suggest that relaxation is an effective strategy for them, even minor ones. If there are no changes in stress, tension or pain, ask if they feel any more relaxed. Sometimes there is not much change if the individual was already relaxed, leaving little room for improvement. Alternatively, relaxation could be such a new experience for them, and change will only happen once they have had a chance to practise more at home.

BOX W3.6 RELAXATION SCRIPT

As we relax, I'm going to ask you to focus on parts of the body in turn, to tense the muscles for a few moments and then relax. In this way, you will learn to notice tension in the body and learn how to let it go. Be careful, and tense your muscle enough to feel tension, but not enough to cause pain. If anywhere feels painful, then reduce the tension or leave it out completely.

Close your eyes if that feels okay, and just let your body relax as much as it can right now. If there's any tension in the body, let it go. Focus on your breathing for a few moments. Notice how, each time you breathe out, the body relaxes automatically.

Now focus on your hands and tense both of your fists. Feel all of the feelings of tension in both hands. Notice what it is like . . . . Good. Now, relax, relax. Just let your hands relax and feel the feelings of relaxation growing in your hands . . . .

Now tense your upper arms by bending your arms and touching each shoulder with a hand. Feel all of the tension in your bicep muscles . . . Hold it . . . Good, now relax, relax. Just let your arms relax back to your sides or lap. Just feel the relaxation developing in your arms. Loose, limp and relaxed. . . .

Now tense your arms by holding them out in front of you straight, like a sleep walker. Feel the tension all the way down your arms. Hold it as you focus on tension . . . Then relax, relax. Let your arms relax down and notice how the feelings of relaxation in the arms are different from tension. Feel how that relaxation feels.

Now tense up all the muscles of your forehead by wrinkling your forehead and focusing on the tension here. Try to feel how that feels, and then let it go and let your forehead relax, imagine it becoming smoother and smoother. And now, relax, relax. Just let your forehead relax.

Now tense up your face by squeezing your eyes tightly closed, wrinkling up your nose, pursing your lips and clenching your jaw. Feel how all of the muscles in your face are tight and tense, and feel what that is like. Hold it . . . Good. And relax, relax the whole face. Let the eyes be closed but lightly, nose smooth, lips and teeth gently parted. The whole of your face loose and relaxed. No tension anywhere.

Now tense up your shoulders by shrugging and focusing on tension in your shoulders and neck. Feeling what tension here is like. Good . . . Now relax, relax. Let your shoulders fall back down and notice how different they feel when relaxed.

Now take a deep breath into your chest. Hold it [2-second pause] and now breathe out. Notice how, as you breathe out, the tension leaves and your chest feels very relaxed, allowing that relaxation to move into your shoulders and back. Now tighten your stomach muscles by pulling them in tightly, and notice what tension is like in the stomach, really feeling how it is. Now relax, relax. Your stomach muscles are letting go . . . notice the sensations that arise when you relax your stomach, and let the breath come in and out freely now.

Now press down hard with your heels into the floor, and feel tension in your legs, from buttocks to feet. Hold it . . . Feel it . . . And now relax, relax. Let your legs and feet really relax. Let yourself enjoy the relaxation.

Now you are feeling very relaxed, and if there is any tension, just let it fade away. Let your mind now move towards a place that for you feels very special and relaxing. Just let the image of a special place come to mind, imagine yourself moving towards it. Perhaps it is a beach, forest, mountain or room. You feel very relaxed there and haven't a care in the world. Look around and notice what you can see, what colours and shapes . . . .

Now listen and notice what you can hear – perhaps a gentle breeze, birds in the distance, water moving . . . .

Now breathe in and notice what you can smell – perhaps flowers or the rain or the smell of home . . . .

Notice what you can feel – what the ground beneath you is like . . . if there is sun or wind on your skin . . . .

This place is just for you, it can be whatever you want it to be, and it is here to help you feel more and more relaxed. Lie back notice how relaxed and contented you can feel. You can stay here as long as you want to, just enjoying this feeling of total relaxation.

Now I will count back slowly from four to one, and when I reach one, you will open your eyes and feel awake, alert and relaxed. . . 4, 3, 2, perhaps gently opening your eyes . . . 1. Now take your time and when you are ready, tell me what that was like for you.

Common difficulties that may arise in relaxation

- *Overtensing, causing strain and pain.* Excessive tensing of muscles is unnecessary. If you notice overstraining or pain is reported, suggest less vigorous tensing body. If there is preexisting pain or injury, it is advisable to avoid tensing that area, and instead it is equally useful to focus on simply relaxing that part of the body.
- *Reports of a wandering mind or frustration in being unable to concentrate.* This is entirely normal. You can help by suggesting that when the mind wanders, it is fine to just notice where the mind has gone to, and then gently bring attention back to the body or the relaxing image. Sometimes people describe a struggle to get rid of tension in the body, which can have a paradoxical effect. This can be reduced by suggesting that there is no need to fight what is in the body, but if tension does not go, to gently let it be there. In this way relaxation can slowly spread around the body on its own.

- *Falling asleep*. This can happen very easily, and for some people, relaxation becomes a useful sleeping aid. However, before using relaxation as just a sleeping aid, it is important to learn the exercises properly. If falling asleep happens all of the time, suggest doing the exercises sitting up, with the eyes open or at a time of day when the person is more awake.
- *Finding the associated feelings strange or uncomfortable*. This can happen if relaxation is a very new experience, and it can include sensations of sinking or floating. It usually fades with practice, but it can be eased by sitting up, having eyes open and doing the exercises for shorter periods of time at first.
- *Struggling to find an imaginary place, or settling on just one image*. Again, this is a common experience, because the mind will tend to wander during the exercise. Sometimes it is easier to think of somewhere well-known and to spend time trying to engage all of the senses, not just vision.
- *Worry that relaxation is a form of hypnotism*. These exercises are not hypnotism; they are just ways of achieving deep relaxation for the body and mind.

Homework following session 3

Give the patient handouts 7 and 9 (and 8 only if you have done problem solving). These summarize information about stress and relaxation, describe the homework tasks and include a relaxation diary. Ensure that they have a CD or can download the audio guide for relaxation exercises (CD tracks 4 and 5) at www.routledge.com/9781138119017.

Homework

- Practise muscular and imagery relaxation every day. As with the breathing, try to schedule in a regular daily slot and complete the relaxation diary in a similar way as you did with the breathing diary. (You can complete the first row based on their ratings of stress, tension and chest pain before and after the exercise they did today.)
- Continue to practise abdominal breathing for 10 minutes every day, and try to use this breathing whenever stress and/or chest pain occur and notice what happens.
- If needed, put into practise your problem-solving plan, or seek help through the identified routes.

Reference

Marks, E.M., & Hunter, M.S. Perception of bodily sensations during stress induction: A survey to inform cognitive behavioural interventions for people with persistent physical symptoms. Unpublished manuscript.

Session 4

Keeping active

Focus your questions on

- How have stress management and relaxation affected chest pain? How does this link to the chest pain cycle and non-cardiac pain?
- Were there any difficulties this week? How can we reduce these?
- What does the patient believe about activity or exercise? Are there other ways of thinking about activity?
- How does keeping active link to the patient's original goals for treatment?

Summary of session 4

1 Open the session with agenda setting and review of homework tasks using relaxation and problem solving (if applicable).
2 Provide education and rationale for keeping active. Tackle common beliefs about activity.
3 Discuss how avoidance of activity can make anxiety and chest pain worse (understanding safety behaviours).
4 Address practical ways of increasing activity.
   a. Setting activity goals (based on values identified in session 1)
   b. Pacing – working up an activity hierarchy in a realistic manner
   c. Avoiding the overactivity/resting cycle.
5 Set homework.

What you will need

- Written agenda for session 4
- Copy of individual's chest pain cycle and original goals
- Handouts 10–13.

Aims of session 4

Session 4 plans a gradual increase in activity and engagement with life, aligned with the patient's original goals. Most people with chest pain will have reduced or stopped activities, particularly exertion or exercise. In some cases, functioning can become extremely limited, usually because the patient believes that activity will trigger chest pain or even cause a heart attack, stroke or death. These beliefs can be modified in treatment first by providing truthful and helpful information about the benefits of activity. Then the patient tests out what happens if they start to do more activity. Finally, they set meaningful, achievable and sustainable goals for the coming weeks and months.

By this point, most patients will have used breathing and relaxation sufficiently to see some improvement in their symptoms. Such improvements usually increase conviction in the accuracy of the biopsychosocial chest pain cycle by demonstrating repeatedly how stress, tension and overbreathing affect chest pain. This may weaken the strength of their beliefs about chest pain being dangerous, malignant or a sign of cardiac disease. It may also give them sufficient confidence to try out new things, such as getting active again.

You can explain that many people with persistent chest pain avoid activity because they are afraid of what might happen. Perhaps their concerns have been reinforced through messages from health-care professionals, other people or the media convincing them that chest pain is a dangerous, cardiac event. And, if one fears they have a heart problem, they will feel at risk of serious harm or death, and thus feel responsible for mitigating this risk, which leads them to reduce activity. However, assessment and treatment so far suggest this is not the case, so it is safe for them to be active with chest pain. Testing this out slowly will allow them to discover that activity does not lead to disaster but instead leads to improved well-being and even reduced chest pain. Some of the comments about keeping active made by our patients are shown in Box W4.1.

BOX W4.1 COMMENTS MADE BY PATIENTS IN OUR CLINIC ABOUT INCREASING ACTIVITY

"I'm glad that I came here and was pushed to do exercise when I was fearful because now I am able to do it."

"Although the pain continues, now I can manage to keep going despite it."

"I know pain comes on when I'm stressed, so I still keep active but now I try to pace myself."

"I've been more active since knowing the pain isn't from my heart and finding that the breathing and relaxation help."

This work is based on evidence that exercise is beneficial both generally and in the case of NCCP (and indeed in the case of diagnosed coronary disease).

Opening session 4

Begin by welcoming the patient and briefly ask how things have been since the last session. Ask how they have managed their homework in general. Before a detailed review, set the agenda together, adding any additional issues the patient mentions, particularly struggles with homework.

> **BOX W4.2 AGENDA FOR SESSION 4**
>
> Review homework: relaxation (muscular, imagery), problem solving, breathing.
> Address the facts about activity and chest pain.
> Discuss how avoiding activity can make chest pain worse.
> Address goals and values for increasing the patient's activity.
> Create an activity ladder.
> Discuss awareness of the overactivity/resting cycle.
> Set homework.
> Address any additional issues that were added to the agenda.

Homework review

Bridge to the last session by addressing how the patient now understands chest pain and how motivated they feel to continue. Check the relaxation diary if the patient has brought it. Consider using these or similar open-ended questions:

- How did you find last week's session? What did you find helpful or unhelpful?
- Did you manage to practise the relaxation exercises last week? What did you notice? When did you use them? Did you try using them in response to difficulty or chest pain? Can I have a look at what you put in your diary? What do you conclude from this?
- Were there any difficulties with the relaxation? What might help?
- Have you been continuing with the breathing exercises? How is it going?

Watch out for information relevant to the chest pain cycle, noting down any new information. It is important to check in with the outcomes of problem solving or signposting. If the plan of action went well, talk about what happened and how they can keep this going or build upon it next week. Difficulties often arise with the problem-solving plan, so you will need to revisit the original plan and see what needs to change. You can either simplify the solution or choose a different one. Alternately, you may need to break down the problem and focus on a smaller issue that is easier to solve. Problems may also arise with relaxation, and common issues are described in session 3. An example is also given in Box W4.3. If issues of finding time to practise arise, you may need to revisit ideas of prioritizing oneself and this treatment, as discussed in session 2.

BOX W4.3 TROUBLESHOOTING PROBLEMS WITH RELAXATION

Sara struggled with imagery because she couldn't think of anywhere and her mind kept jumping from place to place. The therapist explained that this doesn't matter, and it happens quite often. She asked Sara to think of other places which reminded her of being relaxed, such as a holiday in the past or somewhere she goes to where she feels okay. Sara mentioned a local park that she goes to when the weather is nice, and the therapist suggested she could go there to try and get a sense of the place or even keep a picture of it nearby to help her when doing the imagery.

Activity and chest pain: the facts

It is important to acknowledge negative beliefs about activity and potential risks, consider how these might be unhelpful and consider that alternative points of view are possible. It may help to think about how other people respond when the patient has chest pain and how such responses affect the patient. For example, some family members encourage someone to stop exercising or rest when they get chest pain, and some patients may even be bought a wheelchair or domiciliary oxygen.

Research evidence supports the view that regular moderate activity is beneficial, whether you have chest pain or not. Consistent advice (even for people with heart disease who are attending cardiac rehabilitation) is to do regular, moderate activity. After explaining this to the patient (an example of how to do this is in Box W4.4), allow the patient to express any concerns or ask any questions they might have. This work can be supported by handout 10.

BOX W4.4 SAMPLE EXPLANATION ABOUT ACTIVITY AND CHEST PAIN

You've told me that you are less active now because of your chest pain. You've stopped walking to work and you now rely on friends to go to the shops for you. One of the main reasons is because you are worried that exercise might trigger chest pain or even cause a heart attack. In fact, medical advice is the opposite, because activity is good for you.

We know from the tests that your heart is healthy, so exercise poses no danger. In fact, even people with heart disease are advised to remain active. The medical evidence shows that regular, moderate activity is good for your health. It makes you fitter and stronger, lowers blood pressure, reduces the risk of heart disease and other illnesses, and it is great for managing stress and improving mood. Simply helping patients with chest pain reach 75% of their maximum heart rate for 12 minutes on a treadmill can lead to improvements (Jonsbu et al., 2011).

> Avoiding activity has the opposite effect and makes chest pain worse. Your body loses strength and fitness quickly, so after a short period of inactivity, you find it harder to be active. When you try, you probably struggle for breath, which can trigger chest pain, and you might strain your muscles, which can also cause of pain. And think of all the things you are no longer doing and how this makes you feel. If you always avoid activity, you will always worry about what might happen if you do any exercise at all, so you get stuck. This is because you don't get a chance to find out what happens if you test it out.

It is important to discover what each individual really believes about how avoidance works for them. At this point, we sometimes introduce the idea of avoidance as a safety-seeking behaviour or something we do to try and protect ourselves from a perceived risk that is not helpful in the long-run.

For example, people who fear spiders usually believe that spiders will attack and cause harm. In fact, this is rare, and spiders usually run away when approached. People with a fear of spiders will never discover this because they always run away from and avoid spiders. Their perception of the risk posed by spiders becomes very exaggerated. Over time, in severe phobia, the perceived risk grows, and the spider phobic spends much time and energy checking for and avoiding spiders. This can lead to major problems in their lives, and they never have the chance to find out what happens if they don't avoid spiders. The fear of spiders and the belief of the danger posed by spiders is maintained.

For a lighter example, we sometimes tell the story of Vlad, a young man who believes in vampires (see Wells, 1997). To keep himself safe, Vlad goes to bed at night with garlic strung around his neck. He has never seen a vampire, and he concludes that the garlic must be working. What would Vlad have to do to find out whether the garlic is working or whether in fact there are no vampires at all? As with the spider example, Vlad will have to stop his avoidance safety behaviour, go to bed without garlic and see what happens.

In NCCP, the perception of risk is high, yet the actual risk is close to zero. The avoidance behaviour leads to long-term decline in functioning and the patient never manages to test out whether their fears are realistic. Inactivity also leads to a decline in physical condition and can exacerbate issues such as musculoskeletal problems, pain, breathlessness during exertion, stress and low mood. The unfortunate result is that when the patient tries to be active, they may actually be more likely to experience chest pain (from breathlessness, muscle strain or stress), and this will only increase their anxiety and avoidance. The only way in which the individual can reverse this process is to drop the avoidance and safety-seeking behaviours. They need to slowly build up their activity levels. This offers them the chance to find out that activity, even if it triggers chest pain, will not lead to a catastrophic event. Over time, fitness should also increase, reducing the frequency of chest pain triggers.

Why do you want to increase activity? Revisiting goals and values

Refer back to the original values-based SMART goals from session 1; motivation to engage with today's agenda will be enhanced if it is clearly linked to the patient's reasons for treatment. Most people with NCCP have limitations and losses because of it. Today is about recouping these losses. Keeping active doesn't necessarily mean exercising, although this is often involved. Rather, it is about living life in the way one wants. With the patient's original goals list, complete the box on handout 10 (How can I keep active?). Ask the patient to think about how chest pain affects their life and inhibits their actions. You may like to use some of these questions as prompts:

1. What activities is chest pain stopping you from doing?
2. What concerns you have about these activities? (Are these on the chest pain cycle?)
3. How can you find out if your worries or concerns are realistic?
4. What were your original goals for treatment?
5. What are you *already doing* that meets your values, and how can you build on these to move towards your goals?
6. Are there any activities you might be able to start doing right now?

The patient can write the answers down. If they struggle to come up with ideas, the following examples might offer some guidance.

Example: Hassan and taking his son to the park

Hassan's goals for treatment were to understand the cause of chest pain and to be able to take his young son to the park on the weekend. At the start of treatment, he was unable to walk more than the 5 minutes to the bus stop, so he couldn't get to the park (which was a 20-minute walk or a bus ride away). He had noticed a big improvement from using the breathing exercises, and he felt that the chest pain cycle explained what was happening. He therefore felt that increasing his activity would be okay, and he had independently begun to walk more often. His values were focused around his family and spending more quality time with them, which would require being able to walk to and around the park. Over several weeks, he gradually worked up from 5 to 20 minutes walking, which allowed him to get to the park. He then began to kick a ball back and forth, and over time he was able to play football with his son, a goal he initially thought impossible.

Example: Paula and losing weight

Paula's hoped that treatment would reduce chest pain so that she could follow her exercise plan for weight loss. Her doctor indicated this was necessary if she wished to improve fertility. As such, weight loss was closely aligned with fundamental values around family and health. Chest pain had prevented her from doing this before, because she feared it might cause a heart attack. At the start of treatment, she was only walking slowly for short distances. She felt that the best way for her to build fitness was to increase her walking in terms of speed and distance, and we developed a graded plan. As she began to walk more often, she found that her fears about a heart attack were unfounded, and she continued walking even when chest pain occurred. After 3 months, Paula was walking 30 minutes to and from work every day. She felt fitter, she had begun to lose weight and her chest pain was less frequent.

Example: Chaya and going to the synagogue

Chaya's chest pain meant she had stopped seeing friends; she felt unable to go to the synagogue, as she didn't want to burden other people with her problems. Her treatment goals were to get back to normal life (going to the synagogue regularly, volunteering for a charity). By session 4, she could recognize how chest pain was related to stress and grief caused by her husband's death after a long illness. She had initially struggled to set aside time for homework, leading to a discussion about how she habitually put other people's needs first without taking care of herself. By prioritizing her treatment, Chaya had begun to spend 45 minutes each day on breathing and relaxation, with big changes to her chest pain. Increased confidence in her chest pain cycle meant that the pains were no longer interpreted as dangerous and she was able to go out more. Her mood improved when she returned to the synagogue and saw her friends, and her chest pain became even less frequent. By the end of therapy, she had begun to volunteer at a charity shop.

The activity ladder: exercise

You can now both work on completing an activity ladder, for which you will need handout 11 to map out the patient's plan to reach their values-based goals. The term *activity ladder* refers to the ways in which each goal forms a rung. The patient starts at the bottom rung (the easiest one) and slowly works up to the more difficult activities, one at a time.

Activities are only as easy as their most difficult components, so complex or difficult activities need to be broken down into manageable parts. The degree of difficulty is based on a numeric rating given by the patient when asked to identify how difficult a task would be for them to do *right now*. A 0–10 rating scale is used, where 0 means an activity is very easy and 10 means it is very difficult.

Very easy			Quite easy			Quite difficult			Very difficult	
0	1	2	3	4	5	6	7	8	9	10

If something is rated as very difficult (>7) or involves many different steps, then you may prefer to break it down. For example, Fatima relied on her daughter to do her supermarket shopping, and she wanted to be able to do this herself. She rated this activity as at 9 (very difficult). We broke it down into component activities and rated each separately:

- 10-minute walk to the shop = 5
- Push trolley around supermarket = 3
- Pick up items from shelves to put in trolley = 3
- 10-minute walk back from shop carrying bags = 9

Fatima therefore planned to start with the easiest component first using the following plan:

- Drive to and from supermarket with daughter, do shopping alone = 3
- Walk to supermarket with daughter, do shopping, get bus back together = 5
- Walk to and from supermarket with daughter (daughter carrying bags) = 7
- Walk to supermarket and do shopping independently = 10

It can be difficult to acknowledge when something one used to find very easy has become a struggle. It can help to explain that this is normal in NCCP because periods of reduced activity naturally lead to a loss of strength and fitness in the body, making normal activities more difficult. This doesn't have to be a permanent change, and with time and practice, fitness will return and activities will become easier again.

For moderately difficult activities (rated >4), you may need to make modifications; otherwise the patient may become overexerted or fail to complete the plan. A task can be made more manageable by getting help with it, doing it for less time, doing it more slowly and planning in regular rest breaks. Fatima was able to reach her goals by:

- Breaking up the 10-minute walk into two, 5-minute walks, resting for 5 minutes in between
- Doing the walk back with only very light items in the bags at first and building this up slowly

Regular breaks make activity more achievable, as there is a recovery period that reduces the risk of overexertion. Rests should be *planned in advance,* lest they be forgotten or become unhelpful responses to chest pain.

Climbing the ladder

Try to rate every goal in this way so the activity ladder fills up with a range of easier to more challenging activities. Activities on the top rungs of the ladder may seem impossible to achieve now, but over time they should become easier. Movement up the ladder should be slow and steady.

- Once an activity has been done repeatedly for at least a week, re-rate its difficulty.
- If it has become rated as 0 or 1, the patient can move onto another activity.
- Before moving on, re-rate the next activities on the ladder, and choose one that is no greater than 4.
- Moving on too quickly may lead to failure, may increase chest pain or may even lead into an unhelpful overactivity/resting cycle.

The overactivity/resting cycle

If activity levels increase too quickly, there is a risk of risk falling into an unhelpful cycle of doing too much; being overexerted, fatigued or in pain; and having to rest for a period of time. This maintains avoidance and probably causes further physical deconditioning. Figure W4.1 helps illustrate how this cycle can be problematic (it is available for the patient in handout 12).

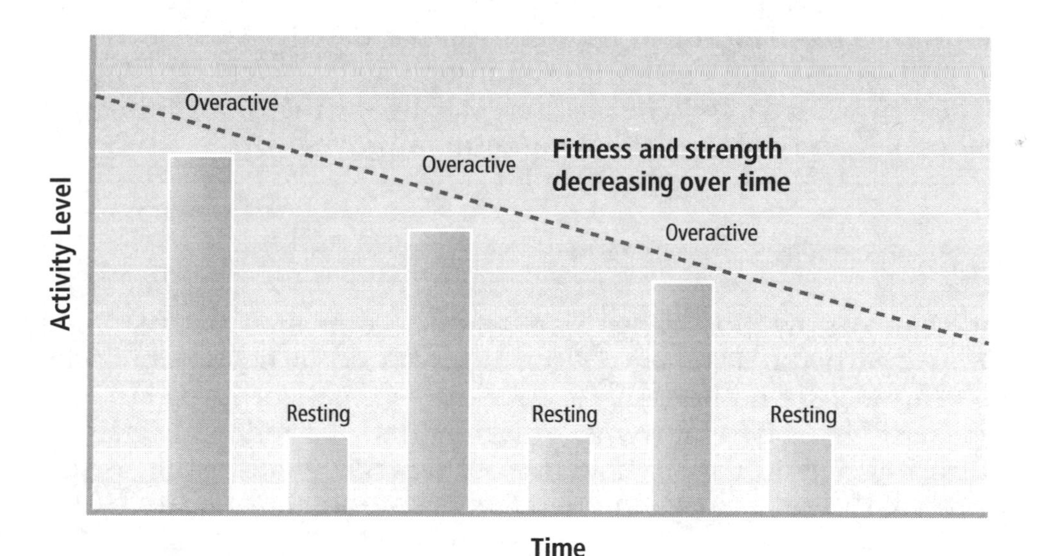

Figure W4.1 Diagram of overactivity/resting cycle

Overactive! On a good day, you might get a burst of energy, feeling ready for anything. When we feel like this, it is tempting to do lots of activity, even more than planned. This can feel good at the time, but overexerting oneself in this way can have consequences the next day.

Rest! After overexerting oneself, the body may be overtired and need to rest. One may then do *less* activity than planned, or no activity at all, for several days.

Falling into the overactivity/resting cycle can delay you from reaching your ideal activity levels. A steady increase will get you there much more quickly. This is because the body loses fitness and strength much more quickly than it builds them up. After a resting period, your body will therefore be less strong than it was before, so when you next try to be active, you may struggle more and get tired more quickly. You may then need to rest again, leading to further loss of fitness and so on.

Pacing

The most successful way to return to increased levels of activity depends upon following a smooth and gradual plan, or *pacing*. It helps to keep going with a regular level of activity without exhausting oneself. Pacing means that even on days when one is feeling more energetic, it is best not to overdo things. Encourage the patient to view the extra energy as something to enjoy that will help them get through the rest of the week. Otherwise they may overexert themselves on a good day and feel over-tired and unable to do even small tasks on the next day.

Pacing means planning and consistently doing the same level of activity each day, regardless of how much energy one has. It begins by figuring out a patient's baseline (the average of their level of activity on a good day and a bad day) and then reducing it by about 20%. This is a baseline level one should begin with doing every day. It often seems surprisingly little, but if they start here they can build up by about 10% per week, or as they feel their body adapting and the activity getting easier. It is critical *not* to increase from the baseline too quickly. If pacing is correct, there should be fewer bad days of feeling exhausted, and more good days.

If the patient overdoes it and needs to rest, encourage them to be kind to themselves but still attempt to do some small activity. Pacing can also be utilized by planning in regular breaks as described previously. It can feel frustrating, particularly if the initial baseline level seems much lower than previous activity levels, but starting at the right point will lead to quicker and more reliable long-term improvement.

Experimenting with activity for homework

We find that by now most patients are ready become more active, based on evidence gathered in support of the biopsychosocial chest pain cycle, and you can just set homework. However, if your patient is too anxious to increase their activity at home, you may find the following helpful in guiding a discussion about how they could try. If your patient is still unable to try this, they may require referral on for high-intensity CBT.

- *Rationale:* What is the patient's rationale for choosing an activity to do (e.g. medical advice for keeping active, values and goals)?
- *Choice:* Can they choose one activity at the lowest end of their ladder and plan it exactly? Schedule when, where and how over the next week.
- *Prediction:* What do they predict what will happen? How will they feel and think? What will happen with chest pain? How they will cope? What will happen next?
- *Doing it:* At home, after doing the activity, the patient will make a note of what actually happened.

- *Conclusions:* They can then compare their predictions to the actual outcomes and reflect on what really happened (you can do this in the next session together). What does this tell them about activity?
- *Troubleshooting:* Some patients may do an activity and still feel very anxious. They may feel that they were only okay because they were using a safety behaviour, for example, monitoring their heart rate, praying, holding on to something or someone when walking. In such cases, they need to try repeating the exercise without this safety behaviour. If the patient has not managed at all, the chosen activity may be too challenging and needs to be made easier, or they may need intensive CBT.

Homework following session 4

Give the patient handouts 10–13 from the session. If you revisited problem solving, you might also give the patient the problem-solving sheet (handout 8). Handout 13 includes the homework list and activity diary.

Homework

- Experiment with using the activity ladder as described. Start with the baseline activity each day if possible. This should be preplanned. Complete the homework diary for each activity done so progress can be monitored.
- Gradually move up the activity ladder, but only when the easiest can be rated as 0 or 1 out of 10. This will take a few days or weeks. It is important not to overdo it.
- Continue to use relaxation and breathing regularly and in response to chest pain.
- Try further problem-solving tasks, if these have been set.

References

Jonsbu, E., Dammen, T., Morken, G., Moum, T., & Martinsen, E.W. (2011). Short term cognitive behavioural therapy for non-cardiac chest pain and benign palpitations: A randomised controlled trial. *J Psychosom Res* 70: 117–23.

Wells, A. (1997). *Cognitive therapy of anxiety disorders: A practice manual and conceptual guide*. New York, NY: John Wiley & Sons.

Session 5

Thinking about chest pain

Focus your questions on

- What has been done with activity? What does this suggest about chest pain?
- What does the patient believe about chest pain now?
- How and why is this different from before?
- How do negative beliefs about chest pain affect emotions and reactions to it?
- Can the patient find more helpful, alternative ways of thinking about chest pain based on what they have discovered so far?

Summary of session 5

1 Open the session with agenda setting and review of homework tasks around activity.
2 Discuss the rationale for why thoughts and beliefs are important in maintaining the vicious cycle of chest pain.
3 Look at common thoughts and beliefs about chest pain and how these are often unhelpful and untrue (cognitive strategies).
4 Challenge thoughts and find more helpful alternatives.
5 Develop a 'helpful thoughts flashcard' to use when chest pain occurs.
6 Discuss how attentional focus makes chest pain worse and how to use distraction.
7 Set homework.

What you will need

- Written agenda for session 5
- Copy of individual's chest pain cycle
- Copy of individual's activity ladder
- Handouts 14–18.

Aims of session 5

Previous sessions mainly focused on behavioural changes (breathing, relaxation and increasing activity) that implicitly challenge a cardiac and biomedical model of chest pain. As a result, by this point many patients tell us that they have already begun to think very differently about chest pain, although some concerns may continue. Session 5 helps to reduce these concerns by explicitly focusing on evidence for and against the patient's beliefs about chest pain. It is therefore essential to identify any outstanding unhelpful thoughts and beliefs. You can then use education, discussion, reflection and cognitive restructuring tasks to reshape these beliefs. The aim is to enable the patient to think about chest pain in a way that is less negative and more realistic, helpful and supportive to pain management.

We have seen how negative thoughts in NCCP are prevalent and are related to social factors, such as the prevalent sociocultural discourse about chest pain and the reactions of other people. Negative thoughts maintain the chest pain cycle because they can fuel anxiety, lead to unhelpful behavioural changes and even directly affect the perception of pain itself. Negative thoughts also change attentional processes. It is natural, if one believes chest pain is a threat, to monitor for signs of that threat, and patients often report paying selective attention to their bodies, looking out for signs of chest pain. Unfortunately, monitoring the body actually makes the patient more sensitive to change and more likely to notice normal fluctuations they would previously have ignored. These minor fluctuations can be misinterpreted as dangerous or abnormal, which feeds back into chest pain cycle. It is possible to interrupt this process by reducing monitoring and learning to direct the attention elsewhere, for example, by using distraction. People with NCCP in our clinic find the cognitive strategies in session 5 very helpful. Some examples of their comments about this are in Box W5.1.

BOX W5.1 COMMENTS MADE BY PATIENTS ABOUT COGNITIVE STRATEGIES

"I feel as if I have more control because I understand the chest pain. Treatment has made me think differently, and so now, when I feel stressed, I know I will be okay."

"Understanding the link to acid reflux calmed me down."

"I found the 'helpful thoughts flashcard' the most useful part of the therapy."

"I thought stress might have caused chest pain but I wasn't sure. Now I know it is the main cause of my pain, because of what you taught me. Knowing this makes me very reassured, and my husband too."

"I'm using distraction when chest pain happens, and keep doing small tasks."

"Now I see the vicious cycle, I can think about the positives, whereas before I only saw the negatives. So it has changed how I think about things. My daughter has just

continued

given birth and now I can see new life as well as the loss, before I'd just have seen the loss [an earlier bereavement]."

"I found it helpful to write down all my symptoms and notice what I think about them and how this makes me feel. Now I can see how the mind creates the vicious cycles and makes it worse."

Opening the session

Welcome the patient and find out about the last week. Set the agenda as usual.

BOX W5.2 AGENDA FOR SESSION 5

Review homework and troubleshoot activity increase.
Discuss how thoughts and thinking patterns affect chest pain, and address common thoughts in chest pain.
Look at the patient's unhelpful thoughts about chest pain and work on developing more helpful ones.
Discuss attention and distraction.
Set homework.
Address any additional items.

Homework review

As always, check in with the homework, and find out what the patient managed to do. If changes were small, try to pull out any improvements as proof of their ability to move towards their goals. If available, look though their activity diary, following up with one or two of these questions:

- How did you find last week's session? Was there anything you found particularly helpful or unhelpful?
- How did you do with your plan to increase your activity? Did anything go very well? Did anything go not so well?
- What did you write in your diary?
- What do you conclude from being able to make this change?
- Are you still using breathing and relaxation exercises? Did they help you cope with the activity at all?

As usual, refer to the patient's chest pain cycle and add any new information. Keep asking open questions to help the patient think about what they have learnt over the last week that supports the biopsychosocial formulation.

Many people struggle with activity homework, particularly when they are working out what the best baseline level is for them. Some overdo it; others don't do enough and lack confidence to follow the plan. It is possible that the activity triggered chest pain, which may have increased fear. Be sure to assess carefully to pinpoint specific barriers that prevented them from keeping to the plan, so that the plan can be restructured for next week. The most common issues with not keeping to the plan are:

- The activity chosen was too difficult. If this is the case, choose an easier activity, or make the activity easier with pacing, support from others or breaking it into smaller parts.
- The patient remains very anxious about chest pain. If this happens, perhaps focus on the cognitive aspects covered in this session before setting up a new activity for homework. You may also need to consider referral on for high-intensity CBT.

If homework has gone well, then you can use this part of the session to plan for next week. Ask the patient to rate the activity again for difficulty. If it has reduced to 0 or 1, they can decide to move up to the next activity on their ladder, providing this is achievable now (i.e. 4 difficulty level). Otherwise, they can slightly increase last week's activity by about 10%, either by doing it for a longer time, taking fewer rest breaks or doing it more intensively.

Why thoughts and beliefs are important

Refer back to the chest pain cycle to highlight the central role of cognitions (thoughts and beliefs) in maintaining chest pain and causing emotional, physical, behavioural and attentional changes. For this reason, today you will be exploring how the patient thinks about their chest pain. You may find the sample explanation in Box W5.3 useful.

BOX W5.3 SAMPLE EXPLANATION FOR WHY TODAY FOCUSES ON THOUGHTS ABOUT CHEST PAIN

Everybody thinks about bodily sensations differently. This depends on factors such as your previous experiences with such sensations, what other people or the media say, or how healthcare professionals have reacted. When one first has a symptom like chest pain, it is normal to think there may be something wrong and it is appropriate to seek medical advice. However, if, after the right tests and medical reassurance negative thoughts continue, they can become very unhelpful. Many people with persistent chest pain tell us that they fear the medical tests have missed some serious underlying problem, and they remain worried and think chest pain is still a sign of something dangerous.

continued

This is not your fault; it is a rational response to what the world tells us about chest pain. For example, if you look up the term chest pain online, you will see hundreds of web pages talking about heart problems and advising you to seek emergency help. Similarly, as the medical system is cautious, the immediate response to chest pain is to do tests that can rule out cardiac disease. These can reinforce the sense of danger. No time is spent discussing alternative explanations for the pain, so you can be left feeling anxious, confused and still believing chest pain is dangerous.

It is important to know that these negative thoughts directly affect how we experience pain. You can see this for yourself. Imagine that two people have headaches. The first person believes the headache is because she is dehydrated, and the second believes he has a brain tumour. Whose headache will feel worse? Clearly, the person who believes he has a brain tumour will feel more scared, have more pain and focus more on the headache than the person who just thinks it is dehydration. The same thing happens in chest pain; just imagine the different experiences of someone who thinks chest pain is caused by cardiac disease, compared to someone who thinks it is acid reflux.

Negative thoughts also affect how we pay attention to some things. Humans (and animals) naturally keep an eye out for potential sources of threat. If you believe that chest pain is threatening, then you will naturally spend more time focusing on your body and looking out for early signs of chest pain. Unfortunately, this makes you more sensitive to changes in the body, and you notice sensations that are just normal, minor fluctuations. This feeds the fear and the chest pain cycle. Like the old adage says, "when you go looking for trouble, you find it!"

So, logically, if negative thoughts about chest pain maintain it, then changing these thoughts should lead to an improvement in chest pain. If you are less worried about chest pain, then it will be less problematic and intrusive.

Common unhelpful beliefs about chest pain

You are probably already aware of the patient's automatic negative thoughts, and you can move directly into the exercise in handout 14. If not, you can explore this by asking the patient to recall a recent, typical chest pain episode. As they remember it, ask the following questions and note their answers:

- What went through your mind last time you had chest pain?
- When you had chest pain, what did you think was causing it? What did you think would happen?
- Did you have any pictures or images about what was going to happen?

Handout 14 lists common beliefs identified by our patients with NCCP. These mostly related to threatening causes, catastrophic consequences and losing control. Explore this with your patient using the table on handout 14, concealing the right-hand column and asking the patient to write down whether each statement is true or false. Then reveal actual answers (based on medical evidence) and compare the two columns. Any discrepancies can be highlighted before moving onto handout 15.

In our clinic, many patients complete the table in handout 14 correctly; they already understand the medical facts. It is still worth doing this exercise and exploring with the patient what has enabled them to understand chest pain in this way, if this has changed because of treatment, and if they will be able to think like this in the future. This is important because it is one thing to be calm and rational about chest pain with your therapist in a session and quite another when you experience severe chest pain on your own.

Thinking more helpfully about chest pain

Treatment should have provided plenty of evidence in support of the biopsychosocial model, which is more helpful than seeing chest pain as a cardiac issue, such as evidence provided from the initial assessment; information gathered about the benefits of abdominal breathing, relaxation and stress management; evidence about the actual consequences of chest pain and evidence they can be active despite chest pain.

This does not mean that all their concerns will have vanished, but it does mean you have the proof required to build a new way of thinking about chest pain. Handout 15 guides you through this. You can both look at the list of common chest pain worries, identify those relevant to your patient, and add any specific concerns. You can decide on which of the more helpful thoughts can be used in place of the worrying thought (again with the patient adding any of their own).

Managing barriers to helpful thoughts

If you need extra support in this, handout 15 includes some tips on how to build up the alternative, helpful thoughts. The patient can rate how strongly they believe a helpful thought is (using a 0 to 10 scale). If an alternative thought has a low rating (i.e. below 7/10), this indicates that the patient has outstanding concerns in a particular area. You can then focus your discussion on this particular belief. Try to find out what prevents them from believing the helpful alternative and what additional evidence or information would help them believe it more strongly.

Discussion can follow the guide on handout 15. You may also like to use some of the following questions to help you to explore the negative thinking in more detail. You may want to note the patient's answers to refer to in the future.

- What stops you from believing (this helpful alternative thought) more strongly?
- What would help you believe this thought more strongly?
- Can you think of any evidence in support of this thought? Prompts:
    - Evidence from test results/doctor's assessment
    - Evidence from triggers of pain and what this might indicate
    - Evidence from what helps pain and what this indicates
    - Evidence that you have some control over your pain using strategies.

- Have your fears about the consequences of chest pain ever happened? If not, why might this be?
- Have you learnt anything over the past few weeks that suggests that your worries about chest pain may not occur?
- Have you learnt anything in the past few weeks that suggests these alternative thoughts might be true and more helpful for you?

Troubleshooting: when there is distress but you cannot identify negative thoughts

Some patients do not report catastrophic beliefs, yet they remain distressed about chest pain. This may be because the patient is not aware of their negative thoughts, or finds them difficult to verbalize. In such cases further exploration is helpful. Ask the patient to tell you about a recent chest pain episode where they felt strong emotions, and try to focus on the thoughts they had at this time. You may then need to ask more probing questions to uncover the meanings of such thoughts. Helpful questions may ask about what the patient fears most or what the worst possible outcome could be. When you have identified a thought about chest pain, you could use some of the following questions to explore in more depth:

- And what does that thought mean to you?
- And if that were the case, what is the worst thing that could happen?
- And if that thoughts was true, what would that mean?
- And then what might happen?

An example of how to use these thoughts is shown in Box W5.4.

BOX W5.4 EXAMPLE OF HOW TO EXPLORE NEGATIVE THOUGHTS IN MORE DETAIL

Mark had noticed some benefit from treatment. He told his nurse therapist that his initial fear that chest pain was caused by his heart had gone, and treatment had successfully broken the link between pain and the heart. However, his chest pain continued and he felt angry about this because he didn't understand why it was persisting. The following is an example transcript of how Mark and his nurse attempted to understand the beliefs underlying his continuing anger and distress.

Nurse: Can you tell me about the last time you got chest pain and felt angry?
Mark: On Tuesday afternoon, after having a difficult meeting with a client.
Nurse: How were you feeling that afternoon?
Mark: I was quite stressed out; we're understaffed and I had loads to do.
Nurse: And then what happened?
Mark: I got a stabbing pain in my chest.
Nurse: Did you notice anything else in your body then?

Mark: Yeah, I was really tense in my shoulders and back and felt quite hot.
Nurse: What emotions did you feel when the chest pain happened?
Mark: I was stressed, and then I got really, really annoyed.
Nurse: Anything else?
Mark: No, I was just annoyed. Angry actually.
Nurse: As you were feeling angry, what thoughts were going through your mind?
Mark: I was like, Oh no! Not chest pain again! This is so unfair!
Nurse: And what is it that made you think it was unfair?
Mark: I have so much to deal with right now, it's not fair I have chest pain too. It should be gone by now.
Nurse: And for what reason do you think it should have gone by now?
Mark: I've been coming here, working hard, doing what you said would help, but I'm still getting it. I understand my heart is okay, so then why hasn't it stopped?
Nurse: And what does it mean to you that the chest pain hasn't stopped?
Mark: Well, obviously the treatment hasn't worked properly.
Nurse: And if that's the case, what might happen?
Mark: That I'll keep getting chest pain forever, and eventually I won't be able to cope.
Nurse: And if you keep getting chest pain forever, what will happen?
Mark: Eventually I'll have to give up because I won't be able to cope.
Nurse: What will you have to give up if you couldn't cope?
Mark: Everything. I'll be back at square one, totally messed up, unable to do what I have to.
Nurse: And then what will be the worst that will happen?
Mark: I'll end up out of a job, and probably out of my home too.
Nurse: So it sounds as if you are still worried about chest pain and what might happen in the future. Your thoughts are that, because you are still getting chest pain, treatment must not have worked, and this means it will all get worse again, and eventually you will end up out of work.
Mark: Yeah, I guess that's right.

Mark and the nurse have uncovered the belief about continuing chest pain that seems to be increasing distress. This is another worrying thought to write on handout 15. They then moved on to replacing the thought with a more helpful alternative.

Nurse: This is a worrying thought for you. Although you're okay now, you think that things will get worse if chest pain doesn't stop completely. Can we talk through this a bit more?
Mark: Okay.
Nurse: What triggered your pain last Tuesday?
Mark: It was that difficult meeting; I guess I was feeling pretty stressed.
Nurse: Looking at your chest pain cycle, can we see why this triggered the chest pain?
Mark: If I get stressed, then I get tense, especially in my neck and shoulders.
Nurse: What did the doctor say about muscular tension here?
Mark: She said that tension made my old shoulder injury feel more painful.
Nurse: And how did that relate to the chest pain?
Mark: She said that sometimes pain from the back can feel like it's in the chest, because of how the nerves are located in the body.
Nurse: And have you noticed anything that suggests this is true?
Mark: I guess so, when my shoulder gets stiff I can feel sore in my chest too, and when I do the relaxation exercises it can help the pain.

continued

Nurse: So how much do you believe the pain is caused by tension, from 0–10?
Mark: It must be true – 9/10.
Nurse: What happened when you tried to use these exercise on Tuesday?
Mark: I didn't try! I was too annoyed and had far too many other things to do.
Nurse: So it sounds like you were under a lot of pressure at this point and it was too difficult to take the time to use the exercises.
Mark: Yeah, this week has been very stressful. I've not done much relaxation at all.
Nurse: And if you began doing it again, what do you think would happen?
Mark: I think it would help. It did before.
Nurse: And what do you think would happen with your chest pain if you began doing more relaxation?
Mark: I'd probably cope better.
Nurse: And if you were coping better, what might this suggest about your thought that treatment has not worked and your chest pain will keep getting worse?
Mark: I suppose that if I keep using the relaxation then I can actually cope. Even though I'm really stressed right now, the chest pain is not as bad as it was before coming here.
Nurse: So what happens if we look at chest pain that way? You have it because you are stressed, but you are still coping right now, and you might cope even better if you do more relaxation. How does that feel? How angry does that make you?
Mark: I'm not so angry. I feel like I'm going to be okay in the future. I still want the chest pain to stop, but it's not the end of the world, it's because I'm so stressed.
Nurse: So that sounds like it might be a more helpful thought, shall we write it down?

At this point, Mark and the nurse write down the more helpful thought on handout 15: "I still get chest pain, because I still get stressed and my muscles get tense. If I do relaxation exercises, I can cope, and I can use these in the future too".

Developing a helpful thoughts flashcard

Helpful thoughts, once identified, have to be *practised repeatedly*. Cognitive changes take time, and the patient needs to rehearse thinking these helpful thoughts so that they replace the automatic negative thoughts. To manage this, the patient develops a helpful thoughts flashcard which summarizes today's discussions. A template for the flashcard and the instructions for use are in handout 16. To be effective, flashcards should be specific to the patient, and the patient completes the blank lines with their own particular causes, consequences and coping mechanisms. The flashcard is then used for homework, with rehearsal and response:

Rehearsal: The patient reads the flashcard repeatedly, several times a day. They can carry it with them or display it in a prominent position at home or work (such as on a door, mirror or computer). Reading the statements repetitively will make this way of thinking more automatic, so helpful thought patterns replace the old, negative thought patterns.

Response: The flashcard is also a coping tool. It is difficult to think helpfully and rationally during a chest pain episode, and anxiety can lead back to negative thoughts. The patient can practise reading the flashcard when chest pain occurs or at times of stress. It is a quick and easy reminder about helpful thinking, which can reduce the tendency to focus on negative thoughts when distressed.

Attentional focus and distraction (optional item)

Handout 17 explores the importance of attentional focus, although it may not be relevant for all patients. If you do not have time to cover this in the session, you can give the handout to the patient to read for homework. For those patients who are still very anxious and tend to monitor their body for chest sensations, this is a useful intervention. You should first explain how selective attention focus feeds the chest pain cycle, and then explain how distraction can interrupt the process. A sample explanation is in Box W5.5, and you may want to use Figure W5.1 to support this description of the vicious cycle of selective attention.

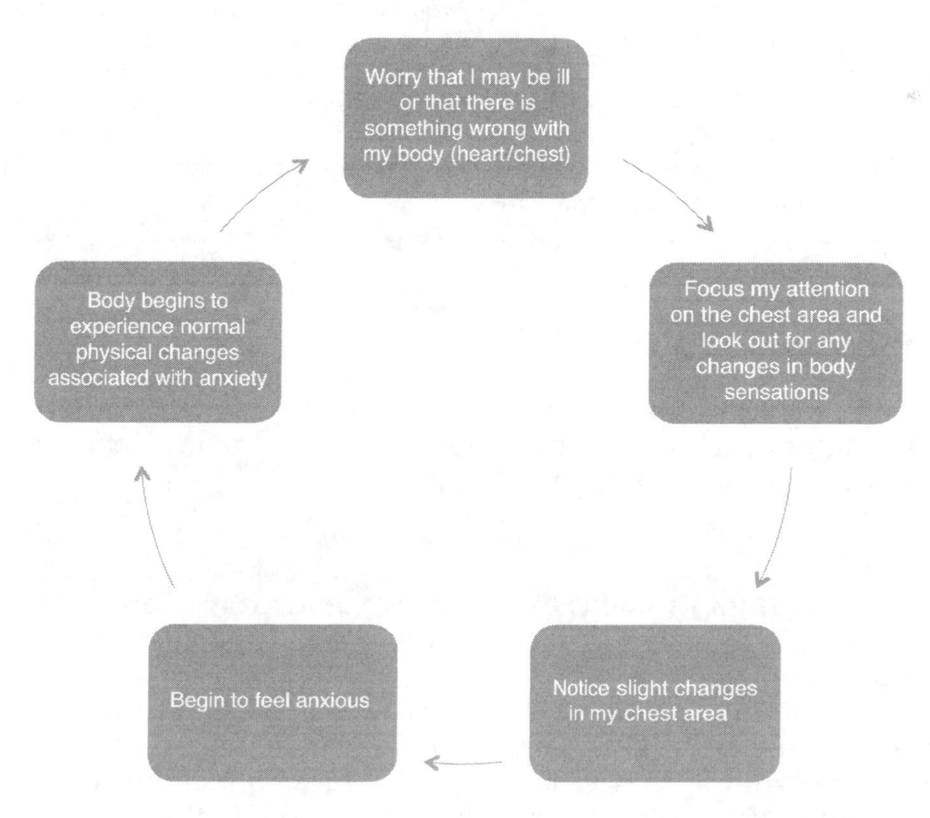

Figure W5.1 How attention feeds chest pain

BOX W5.5 EXAMPLE DESCRIPTION ABOUT DISTRACTION AND CHEST PAIN

If we feel under threat or anxious about something, then it is normal to focus our attention on it. This keeps us alert to possible danger, such as looking out for traffic when we are crossing a road. Sometimes we focus on a possible danger over a much longer period of time. For example, if we are worried that we are ill, we may spend a lot of time focusing on sensations in our body. This can cause problems.

Let's try this out with a little experiment. Spend the next 2 minutes fully focusing on your left leg. Really pay attention to what is happening in your left leg. *[After two minutes:]* What do you notice? What sensations are there now? Do you feel anything in your left leg that you weren't aware of before? What do you think would happen if you kept focusing your attention on your left leg for a whole hour? And what might happen if you began to worry that there was something wrong with these sensations or with your leg? Most people find that they begin to feel more in their leg. If they start to worry, this can feel strange and or unpleasant. In chest pain, this process has been happening to you for a long time, possibly months or even years.

Paying attention to something makes us more aware of the details of it. The body continually has different sensations happening all of the time. This is normal, and we usually ignore these sensations and pay them no attention. However, if we are worried about a particular sensation, this changes. We begin to spend more time focusing on the body, monitoring for sensations, and so we notice them more. This can cause anxiety, which itself can lead to more physical sensations.

It is possible to reduce how much attention you pay to the body. You can practise this whenever you notice yourself monitoring your body or chest. Remind yourself why this is unhelpful and then choose to focus your attention elsewhere. It helps if you can have a predetermined plan or distraction to focus on. So let's think of an activity or mental exercise you find engaging, such as reading, listening to music, thinking about a pleasant memory, doing a puzzle or mental arithmetic or talking to someone. We can make a note of these on your handout, and next time find yourself focusing on your chest, decide to focus on this activity instead.

Homework following session 5

Give the patient handouts 14–18, including any notes taken on them today. Handout 18 summarizes homework. Summarize the relevant homework tasks with your patient.

Homework

- Use the helpful thoughts flashcard by reading it regularly (rehearsal) and when chest pain occurs (response). Follow the instructions given in the handout.
- Use distraction to reduce selective attention and monitoring. (If this was covered in today's session, they should practise the activities identified. If not, they can simply read through handout 17.)
- Continue to work up the activity ladder. Follow the plan that you discussed when reviewing homework today. Remember that you will only increase activity if your current level is rated as 0 or 1 out of 10

in terms of difficulty. If the task is still more difficult than this, keep going with the same activity as last week.

- Continue to use breathing and relaxation regularly, if possible, and also in response to chest pain. If one technique is particularly helpful or one is not helpful at all, choose to continue with just one exercise. You may also find that you can move onto using the shortened relaxation exercise (CD track 5) if they feel confident in the longer one. This is relaxation only (no tensing stage), so it can be useful to do when out and about or in public.

Session 6

Review and maintenance

Focus your questions on

- How has changing thinking affected the patient's experience of chest pain?
- Review treatment overall. What has changed? What has not changed? What was helpful or unhelpful?
- Review value-based goals, and look forward. What are the patient's plans for the future? How can they maintain or develop any improvements?

Summary of session 6

1. Open the session with agenda setting and review of homework tasks of helpful thinking and continuing with activity.
2. Reflect on what has been learnt in therapy and what has been particularly helpful and unhelpful, with reference to:

   a. Biopsychosocial assessment and other causes of chest pain
   b. Understanding the vicious chest pain cycle
   c. Paced, abdominal breathing
   d. Understanding stress, relaxation and stress management
   e. Keeping active and pacing
   f. Thinking about chest pain in a more helpful way.

3. Look at the original goals and seeing if these have been achieved.
4. Measure change on questionnaires.
5. Develop a maintenance plan to keep the positive changes going, minimize barriers and cope with setbacks.
6. Communicate with other health professionals.
7. What additional support can be accessed now or in the future, if required? Discuss how to decide when this is necessary (e.g. if other health problems are detected).

What will you need

- Written agenda for session 6
- Questionnaires (in Appendix 2)
- Helpful thoughts flashcard from last week
- Individual's chest pain cycle
- Individual's initial goals
- Individual's initial questionnaire scores and chest pain diary
- Handout 19 (review and maintenance plan).

Aims of session 6

The sixth and final session draws together all of the work you have covered, revisiting the biopsychosocial CBT model of non-cardiac chest pain and reflecting on what changes have been made and the consequences of such changes. This requires referring back to the original goals and questionnaires. The session revolves around the completion of handout 19 (Review of progress and plan for maintaining positive changes). The patient keeps this to remind them of the issues covered during treatment. The handout provides the structure for the session. Throughout, try to encourage open discussion so the patient can give honest feedback and alert you to any outstanding issues.

The end of a therapeutic relationship can provoke mixed feelings, and part of today's session should address this directly. Feelings for you both may include a sense of achievement, success or relief. The patient may have concerns about losing support from you or your team and having to continue alone. If treatment has been unsuccessful, there may be a sense of failure, disappointment or even anger. If there are outstanding issues, you will need address these and consider whether the patient may need to access further input elsewhere.

Opening session 6

In the few minutes before the session, you can ask the patient to complete the questionnaires (found in Appendix 2) that they did at assessment (it will save you some time if this is done before the session starts). You can then set the agenda together, adding any additional issues as necessary.

BOX W6.1 AGENDA FOR SESSION 6

Review homework on helpful thoughts and distraction techniques (if used).
Review overall progress, to include the following:
- Compare current levels of chest pain to distress to pre-treatment levels (including questionnaires), and link to goals.
- Review treatment, consider helpful and unhelpful aspects.

continued

Discuss maintenance of changes.
  Set goals and make a maintenance plan.
  Address dealing with setbacks.
End the session and say goodbye.
How to access further help if required.
Address any additional items.

Homework review

Find out how much the patient has been able to use the cognitive strategies from last week. Important points to check on are whether the patient managed to use the flashcard (both rehearsal and response) and how this affected their experience. If they have not used the helpful thoughts, find out what prevented this. Examples of issues with cognitive strategies include the following:

- The homework seemed unnecessary because chest pain had not recurred.
- The patient did not think the strategies would work.
- The patient did not believe the new thoughts.

In any case, regular rehearsal is a way of maintaining long-term change and making helpful thinking patterns more automatic (and unhelpful thinking patterns less automatic). If they are sceptical about the new thoughts, you may need to use the rest of the session to review the treatment as a whole with a particular focus on developing new alternative thoughts that are more meaningful to the patient.

Doing the therapy review

The rest of the session follows handout 19, which the patient can fill in as you talk through each question. Before you begin, collect in the questionnaires that the patient did before today's session.

Goals and changes

Ask the patient to recall how they were before the assessment and what their original goals for treatment were, referring to the original goal sheet if necessary. Keep in line with the CBT model by asking about changes in *thoughts, emotions* and *behaviours* around chest pain. For example, if the goal was to manage chest pain better, how has this happened? Are they thinking more helpfully about it? Do they feel less distressed? Are they seeking help less often? Is chest pain interfering less with life? Are they keeping more active?

Compare pre-treatment questionnaire scores to their questionnaire scores today. This is a standard way to measure improvement in chest pain, and comparison to the baseline will show you both the magnitude of change and whether any issues are outstanding.

Review of treatment

If there have been any positive changes, it is important to find out what interventions the patient believes were instrumental to this, because these are probably what will help them to stay well in the future. The chest pain cycle can help guide you through this, identifying whether thoughts, emotions, behaviours, social factors or a mixture of these played the most important roles. Alternatively, the patient may identify something else that was important to them.

As best as you can, encourage honest feedback, because this will help the patient focus in on how to stay well. Similarly, encourage the patient to take notes so they can keep a reminder of therapy after your work has finished. You will probably already be aware of what the patient found helpful and unhelpful, and if necessary you can make suggestions, although it is best to elicit the patient's point of view if possible. When a strategy is identified as helpful or unhelpful, try to explore *why* they think this and how it links to the chest pain cycle. If you can, include everything covered in treatment:

- Understanding what causes my chest pain – that it is not my heart and is not dangerous
- Understanding thoughts, emotions, behaviours and the vicious chest pain cycle
- Learning abdominal, paced breathing
- Understanding stress and learning relaxation skills
- Problem solving and assertiveness
- Testing out and increasing my activity in a graded and paced way
- Learning how to think more helpfully about chest pain.

Both difficulties and successes need to be acknowledged. If some approaches were unhelpful or irrelevant, then the patient may not need to continue with these in the future. For example, some of our patients find the relaxation exercises ineffective, others are not able to fully understand and use abdominal breathing, and others do not meet their activity goals by the final session.

Sometimes this review session can lead you to discover new solutions. For example, patients who found no benefit from relaxation may decide to spend more time on using breathing exercises. Individuals who could not master abdominal breathing may decide to focus on slowing down and paying attention to the breath without having to change it (a technique of mindfulness meditation). Those struggling with activity may decide that their immediate expectations are too high and settle on goals that are more moderate in the short and medium term.

A common issue that arises in the review is having struggled to find time and space to complete the homework tasks. Ways of managing this were discussed in session 2, with a particular focus on motivation and being able to prioritize one's own needs and well-being before other demands. You may find it helpful to revisit this discussion today. You can also help the patient to explore the differences between the times that they managed to do the homework tasks and the times when they did not. This usually the benefits from using the strategies, and they may like to consider how they can implement this in the future.

How to access further help if needed

Not everyone will improve with this treatment. Some people will struggle to make changes and will remain anxious or uncertain about chest pain. This is more likely when there are other significant issues present, such as comorbid mental health issues, physical illnesses and/or challenging, unresolved social problems (e.g. homelessness, asylum status, ongoing court case). Assessment should have identified these issues already, but they may only come to light later on in treatment. If this happens, you will probably have to discuss with your team and/or supervisor how to manage the situation. Options may include referral to local services or the GP. Some examples from our clinic are shown in Box W6.2. A list of resources is provided at the end of the book, if patients need more help or information.

It is important to discuss why treatment may not have been successful, particularly if the patient feels disheartened or believes you, they or CBT has failed. Alternative explanations may be less blaming:

- Perhaps now was not the right time for the patient to have treatment, especially if there are many other demands in their life that need to be resolved first.
- Perhaps the patient did not have enough time to practise all of techniques enough to see a difference yet.
- Perhaps the patient is too distressed to use the strategies such as relaxation or breathing at the moment, but in the future this may become easier, if other sources of distress recede (e.g. for comorbid mental or physical health problems).
- The guided self-help is low intensity. For some people this may not be sufficient, and high-intensity CBT could be helpful in the future.

If chest pain remains and you are unsure why, then it is recommended that this is discussed within your team. You may wish to consider the possibility that an organic cause was not identified at assessment. As outlined in Chapter 7, assessment should already have been completed, ideally with a cardiologist, and cardiac causes should have been excluded. On very rare occasions, the history may change over successive visits, and this could indicate a need for further investigation. This decision requires discussion with the cardiologist in the first instance and prior to your final session.

BOX W6.2 EXAMPLES OF WHEN MORE HELP IS REQUIRED AFTER THE FINAL SESSION

Francisco had lost three members of his family over the past few years, but he had been so busy looking after the rest of his family he had not had a chance to grieve. He found that the treatment helped at first and the frequency of his chest pain had reduced. As he spent more time sitting still with the breathing and relaxation exercises, he noticed he was thinking a lot about the people he had lost. He had started to feel sad most of the time. He wanted to have some help with this, so he was referred to a bereavement counselling service.

Sarah reported that her chest pain was occurring less, but now she was feeling more worried about her headaches. She feared that these might be a sign of a terrible illness, despite her GP requesting appropriate tests and being able to reassure her that these were normal. On discussion, Sarah explained how she had always worried about different aspects of her health before the chest pain (something she had not mentioned before). We discussed how recurrent anxiety about health could mean that she was experiencing health anxiety. She agreed to a referral to a local psychological therapy service for further assessment and CBT.

Bobby had found little benefit from treatment. He still struggled to go out, still felt anxious and was having chest pain quite frequently. In his assessment, Bobby had disclosed that he had been abused in the past and was still affected by traumatic memories about this. He had been offered treatment in the clinic because he wanted to focus specifically on chest pain and nothing else. The clinical psychologist had worked with Bobby using mostly the guided self-help approach. Bobby found that the breathing exercises enabled him to cope better with his traumatic memories as well as his chest pain. In the final session, he felt as if he might benefit from more therapy which would help him tackle his traumatic memories more directly, so we wrote to the GP to suggest he be referred to a traumatic stress service.

Maintenance plan

It is now time to look to the future and your patient's plans for the coming weeks, months and years. If treatment has been very successful, the plan may simply be about maintaining their current state or moving to new goals. If treatment has been less successful, the patient may feel that there are outstanding goals to meet, and you can think of ways to plan for this.

Try to keep in mind the patient's values and original goals, and try to make any future goal setting SMART (specific, measurable, achievable, realistic and time-limited). In developing a maintenance plan, the patient can map out interim goals to meet on their journey towards more ambitious goals. For activity-related goals, remember to think about grading and pacing.

Example

Mary had reached her original goals by the end of treatment. She was less frightened by chest pain, seeing her friends every week and attending the church choir. Her confidence had grown, and by the end of therapy she had identified a new goal: she wanted to return to work. In developing her maintenance plan, we mapped out how Mary could move towards this new goal. She had been working as a teaching assistant with a view to doing teacher training for primary school before her chest pain started, and she still wanted to teach. We discussed how this was a long-term goal that required her to achieve a number of interim goals first. Mary developed the following plan: (1) find part-time volunteer work; (2) find work as a teaching assistant; (3) find out more about the requirements for teacher training; (4) apply for teacher training.

Handout 19 includes a post-therapy maintenance plan where the patient can list their specific goals (short, medium and long term) and identify specifically when, where and how these will be done. For example, someone who simply wishes to maintain their current status and who has benefitted particularly from the breathing and activity ladder might make a plan as shown in Table W6.1.

Table W6.1 Example of how a maintenance plan could be completed

	Goal: breathing	*Goal: activity*
What do I plan to do?	Keep using my breathing exercises	Keep working up my activity ladder until I can walk for 45 minutes without stopping
When do I plan to do it?	Every morning before work and whenever I get chest pain	Every week, in the morning or evening
Where do I plan to do it?	For 10 minutes at home, and then wherever I am when chest pain occurs	On my way to work or on the way home
How often do I plan to do it?	At least once every day, regardless of how I feel	Four times a week; currently managing 15 minutes a day, I will build this up by 5 minutes every 2 weeks

Setbacks

Life is unpredictable and setbacks happen. Preparing for setbacks will minimize their impact and the risk of relapse. The questions on handout 19 guide you through recognizing and coping with setbacks. Some common issues that may help with this are laid out next.

What might lead to a setback or be a barrier to maintaining or making changes?

It may be more difficult to keep going with new strategies without the support of a therapist. In order to stay well, the patient needs to find their own ways of staying motivated. Help them to consider what might get in the way of keeping things going, such as lack of time, feeling better or worse. Interruptions and unexpected stressful events or illness may cause setbacks. For example, how might someone cope with a chest infection that causes respiratory problems and triggers chest pain?

What are the indicators of a setback?

Obviously, an increase in chest pain frequency, severity or intrusiveness indicates a setback. However, there may be subtler changes or warning signs that a setback is approaching. It is easier to cope with a setback if it is caught before a major relapse happens. Patients can think about what early warning signs might alert them, such as:

- Emotional indicators such as feeling stressed, anxious or down.
- Behavioural indicators, such as avoidance of activity, social withdrawal, increased help-seeking.
- Cognitive indicators, such as increased worry about their health
- Social indicators and changes that friends or family might notice; perhaps these people can be recruited help the patient notice important changes.

How can I manage setbacks?

It is best to have a pre-determined strategy for managing setbacks. When warning signs are noticed, the patient can then have a clear plan of action to follow. This might include:

- Reviewing treatment notes
- Using helpful strategies (relaxation, breathing exercise, problem solving)
- If the setback worsens, they can speak to a supportive friend about how they are feeling or ask for help from their GP.

How can I minimize the risk of setbacks?

Whatever worked in the past will probably work in the future. Encourage patients to keep going with helpful strategies. Patients can set regular review sessions to look over handouts from therapy, and we recommend setting aside 1 hour each month for a self-therapy session. This gives the patient an opportunity to check in with their progress, reflect on how they are coping now and stay motivated.

Communicating with other health professionals

Write a letter to the GP or relevant health professional that briefly summarizes therapy and the patient's plans following discharge. You may like to outline what guided self-help treatment covered, how the patient benefitted and if outstanding issues require follow up. You may wish to reiterate that assessment has ruled out underlying cardiac risk at this point and offer the alternative explanation for chest pain. Some patients may have multiple symptoms (e.g. stress-related issues, IBS, headache, other pain) that might continue despite your treatment.

Biopsychosocial assessment will have excluded coronary disease at this time. However, new symptoms could develop in the future. It is important to communicate to the patient that recurrence of chest pain is possible, and it can be managed using the strategies from treatment. The only caveat is if new symptoms develop that are clearly different (e.g. if chest pain is triggered by something new or feels very different), then seeking medical advice would be appropriate.

Ending

Find out how the patient feels about having their last session and moving forward. If possible, give the patient enough time to express how they feel. You can acknowledge that mixed feelings are normal. Most patients will derive benefit from the CBT, but common reactions to ending treatment include the following:

- Feelings of success or achievement, particularly if goals have been achieved.
- Relief, particularly if therapy has been costly in terms of time, energy and money.
- Sadness or disappointment if goals have not been reached or chest pain continues and if the loss of a supportive relationship is difficult.
- Anxiety and uncertainty about whether treatment effects will last after therapy.

You can acknowledge that CBT is a challenging process and that you have seen and appreciated how much effort and hard work they have put into therapy. If a patient was sceptical at first yet managed to do the treatment, you could reflect on their ability to remain open to trying out new suggestions and how this enabled them to change.

Reinforce positive changes and achievements, however small, and that these changes can grow if they keep going with the strategies and plans. This can be framed in a way that is encouraging but without pushing themselves too hard. The message here is one of self-care and of learning to understand what they need to take care of themselves and to give themselves permission and time to do so.

If possible, you may like to schedule a booster session in 3 or 6 months as a way of helping long-term motivation. In evaluating our clinic, we followed up with patients at 3 and 6 months after assessment. Almost all of those reporting improvement by the end of treatment had maintained or furthered this by follow up. This was associated with changes in thinking more helpfully about the causes and consequences of chest pain.

Homework following session 6 (and for the future)

Homework

Give the patient a copy of their completed maintenance plan. Homework for the final session refers to what the patient can do to maintain their gains over the coming weeks and months. Summarize the patient's plan and if appropriate, make suggestions about what other patients with NCCP have found helpful:

- Follow the maintenance plan by using the most helpful parts of treatment identified in the review of treatment.
- If future goals have been set, begin to work towards these in a graded way. Keep going up the activity ladder if there are still outstanding goals to achieve here.
- Set up a monthly self-therapy session where you spend an hour reviewing handouts or notes from therapy, remembering what has been learnt, reflecting on your progress and planning for the next month.

Section 3

Further resources

Information on chest pain

American College of Gastroenterology: Offers an overview of NCCP and how it relates to gastro-oesophageal and other non-cardiac causes, and how these can be treated.
www.patients.gi.org/topics/non-cardiac-chest-pain

National Health Service (NHS): Provides further information about chest pain and common causes, both cardiac and non-cardiac. There are specific pages on common causes of chest pain including gastro-oesophageal reflux, musculoskeletal problems, and anxiety and panic attacks.
www.nhs.uk/Conditions/Chest-pain

NHS Inform: Offers quality-assured health information. There is comprehensive information about the types of interventions that patients may have received because of chest pain (for example, angiography, EEG, aortic valve).
www.nhsinform.co.uk

British Heart Foundation: Registered charity for people seeking information and advice, as well as for health professionals.
www.bhf.org.uk

Lyndon Place
2096 Coventry Road
Sheldon, Birmingham, UK B26 3YU
Tel: +44 (0) 300 330 3311

General health and well-being

NHS Live Well: Offers health and well-being advice with real stories, online assessment and advice about keeping healthy and becoming more active.
www.nhs.uk/LiveWell

Accessing psychotherapy

Improving Access to Psychological Therapy (IAPT): Information about accessing psychological therapy services.
www.iapt.nhs.uk

To find out specific services local to you, and how to access these (either via GP or self-referral), enter your town or postcode at the following web address: www.nhs.uk/service-search/counselling-nhs-(iapt)-services/locationsearch/396.
British Psychological Society: Represents psychologists in the UK.
www.bps.org.uk/psychology-public/find-psychologist/find-psychologist

1 Regent Place
Rugby, Warks, UK CV21 2PJ
Tel: +44 (0) 870 443 5252
Fax: +44 (0) 870 443 5160
bac@bac.co.uk

British Association for Behavioural and Cognitive Psychotherapy: Responsible for the accreditation and training for CBT therapists in the UK and Ireland. There is an online register of accredited CBT therapists.
www.babcp.com

Imperial House
Hornby Street
Bury, Lancashire, UK BL9 5BN
Tel: + 44 (0) 161 705 4304

Mental health and self-help tools

Moodjuice: Offers help and support to people with difficult thoughts, feelings and behaviours. The website offers a variety of self-help guides for various conditions including depression, stress, anxiety, panic and problems with sleep. The site was developed within the NHS Forth Valley in association with the Adult Clinical Psychology Service.
www.moodjuice.scot.nhs.uk

Northumberland, Tyne and Wear NHS Foundation Trust: UK-based health and disability trust. From their website you can download CBT based self-help guides for different conditions including anxiety, panic, anger, obsessions and compulsions, and bereavement.
www.ntw.nhs.uk/pic

Royal College of Psychiatrists: Offers readable, user-friendly and accurate information about mental health problems and how to recognize signs and symptoms. It also includes helpful signposting to relevant services.
www.rcpsych.ac.uk/healthadvice.aspx

MIND: Mental health charity that offers information on many topics on mental health. There is information about symptoms, causes, treatments and support for mental health problems, and there are personal stories and lists of contacts.
www.mind.org.uk

Unit 9, Cefn Coed Parc
Nantgarw, Cardiff CF15 7QQ
Info line: +44 (0) 300 123 3393
info@mind.org.uk

The Samaritans: Offers emotional support for anyone in a crisis, 24 hours per day. It can be accessed online, by phone or in person.
www.samaritans.org.uk

10 The Grove
Slough, UK SL1 1QP
Helpline: +44 (0) 845 790 9090
Fax: + 44 (0) 175 381 9004
jo@samaritans.org.uk

Turn2me: Online community that offers support from peers and professionals to people with anxiety and depression. There are online CBT tools, blog posts, podcasts and informative articles.
www.turn2me.org

1 Pendlebury
Hamworth
Bracknell, Berks, UK RG12 7RB

No Panic: Offers information about anxiety-related difficulties. The website includes information leaflets that can be downloaded.
www.nopanic.org.uk

Jubilee House
74 High Street
Madeley
Telford, Shropshire TF7 5AH
Helpline: +44 (0) 844 967 4848
Tel: :+44 (0)195 268 0460
admin@nopanic.org.uk

Other support

Relate: Offers relationship counselling.
www.relate.org.uk

Premier House, Carolina Court, Lakeside
Doncaster DN4 5RA
Tel: +44 (0) 300 100 1234

Carers UK: Offers information and advice on all aspects of caring.
www.carersuk.org

Carers UK: 20 Great Dover Street, London SE1 4LX
Carers Wales: Unit 5, Ynys Bridge Court, Cardiff CF15 9SS
Carers Scotland: The Cottage, 21 Pearce Street, Glasgow G51 3UT
Carers' line: +44 (0) 808 808 7777

Cruse Bereavement Care: Provides support services for people who have been bereaved.
www.cruse.org.uk

Cruse Bereavement Care
P.O. Box 800
Richmond, Surrey TW9 1RG
Helpline: +44 (0) 808 808 1677
Central Office Administration: +44 (0) 208 939 9530

Divorce Support Group (DSG): Provides local support groups and individual support. It is run by professionals and designed to help people cope with the impact of divorce and separations.
www.divorcesupportgroup.co.uk

Tel: + 44 (0) 844 800 9098
mail@divorcesupportgroup.co.uk

Mindfulness

Be Mindful: Offers information about mindfulness, an online mindfulness course and contact details for mindfulness teachers.
www.bemindful.co.uk

The Oxford Mindfulness Centre and Bangor Mindfulness Centre for Research and Practice: Both have information about mindfulness and how to learn more about it. There are links to good practice guidelines and lists of reliable resources and research.
www.oxfordmindfulness.org
www.bangor.ac.uk/mindfulness

Appendix 1

Invitation to attend the chest pain clinic

This leaflet provides more information about how the chest pain clinic can help people who are experiencing persistent chest pain that is not related to the heart.

What is chest pain? Chest pain can be a sign of heart disease, but for most people it is due to other, less serious causes. This type of chest pain is often called *non-cardiac chest pain,* which means the chest pain is not caused by heart disease. Three-quarters of patients who attend a rapid access chest pain clinic are found to have this type of chest pain. This diagnosis can be reassuring; but, whatever the cause, the chest pain is real and can be helped by a range of treatments.

What causes chest pain? Chest pain is very common and can have several causes. All pain is influenced by a combination of physical, psychological and social factors. Once heart disease has been excluded (which it will have been if you are treated at our clinic), then none of the other causes are medically serious. So you can safely return to living a normal life without chest pain limiting what you do.

- *Physical factors that can cause chest pain:* Pain and tension in the muscles between the ribs; pain in the chest wall from strains or tears in the muscles or ligaments; breathing too fast or over-using the chest to breathe; spasm, tightening or inflammation of the oesophagus (the food pipe); digestive causes such as ulcers causing pain that seems to come from your chest; pain from nerves in the neck or back.
- *Psychological factors can influence chest pain:* Stress and chest pain lead to changes in thinking, emotions and behaviour, for example, in how one reacts to and copes with pain. The stress from both chest pain and from other concerns in life can make chest pain worse. This affects well-being, making it harder to cope with pain.
- *Social factors that can affect chest pain:* Chest pain can make it harder to work, manage responsibilities or other activities. If other people are concerned about your health, this may make you more anxious or dependent. Over time, this can lead to changes in relationships and quality of life.

A biopsychosocial model of non-cardiac chest pain

What is the chest pain clinic? Our chest pain clinic helps people who have had an assessment in cardiology and have been found to have chest pain that is not caused by a problem with the heart. We aim to

- Ensure that all other causes of your chest pain have been considered.
- Help you find ways to manage the pain and improve your general well-being.

There is often a physical cause for chest pain that is *not* from the heart. These physical causes often interact with psychological and social factors, so we think the most useful way to help people with chest pain is to think about the whole picture. This is called a *biopsychosocial approach.* Our approach is evidence-based and has already helped many people with persistent chest pain.

What happens at the appointment? You will meet with a therapist who will ask you more about your chest pain and how it affects your life, whether you have had any other problems with your health that might be relevant, and if these have been treated. We will discuss what factors (physical, psychological and social) affect your chest pain. You will have time to ask questions and be involved in your treatment plan, which will be based on recent research on how to best help people to manage chest pain.

How long will the appointment take? The first appointment will take about 1 hour.

What do I need to bring with me? Please bring a list of all the medicines you are taking, including any medicines you have bought over the counter or herbal remedies. Please fill out the enclosed questionnaires on the day of your appointment and bring these, too.

Will there be any follow-up appointments? Probably; it will depend on the treatment plan we agree on. These follow up appointments will last for 30–50 minutes.

Is there anything I can do to help myself? There are several things you can do that can really make a difference. We will go through these in more detail at your appointment.

Appendix 2

Assessment tools

Frequency of chest pain (from Chambers et al., 2014)

How often do you currently have a chest pain/sensation (check one)?

- All the time
- Several times a day
- About once a day
- Two or three times a week
- About once per week
- About once every 2 weeks
- About once a month
- Less than monthly
- Rarely (less than four times per year)
- Never

Chest pain severity and problem ratings (from Chambers et al., 2014)

For each question, circle one number on each scale in Figure A2.1a that best applies to you now.

SEVERITY OF CHEST PAIN (score 0–10)
How **severe** is your chest pain, on average?

1 ____ 2 ____ 3 ____ 4 ____ 5 ____ 6 ____ 7 ____ 8 ____ 9 ____ 10
Mild Agonizing

INTERFERENCE OF CHEST PAIN (score is the average of scales a, b and c)

a) How **distressing** is your chest pain, on average?

1 ____ 2 ____ 3 ____ 4 ____ 5 ____ 6 ____ 7 ____ 8 ____ 9 ____ 10
No distress Extreme distress

b) How much does your chest pain **interfere** with everyday life?

1 ____ 2 ____ 3 ____ 4 ____ 5 ____ 6 ____ 7 ____ 8 ____ 9 ____ 10
No interference Extreme interference

c) How much of a **problem** is your chest pain for you?

1 ____ 2 ____ 3 ____ 4 ____ 5 ____ 6 ____ 7 ____ 8 ____ 9 ____ 10
No problem Extreme problem

Figure A2.1a

Cardiac belief ratings

For each question, circle one number on each scale in Figure A2.1b that best applies to you now.

NEGATIVE BELIEFS ABOUT CHEST PAIN (Score a and b separately)

a) When you have a chest pain/sensation, do you think you may be about to **have a heart attack**?

1_____2_____3_____4_____5_____6_____7_____8_____9_____10
No, not at all Yes, definitely

b) Do you believe that the chest pain/sensation means that you **have a serious heart condition**?

1_____2_____3_____4_____5_____6_____7_____8_____9_____10
No, not at all Yes, definitely

Figure A2.1b

Depression

Over the last 2 weeks, how often have you been bothered by any of the problems listed in Table A2.1? Please circle the number that best applies to you for each question.

Table A2.1 Patient Health Questionnaire 9 (PHQ 9) to measure levels of depression

PHQ – 9	*Not at all*	*Several days*	*More than half the days*	*Nearly every day*
1 Little interest or pleasure in doing things	0	1	2	3
2 Feeling down, depressed or hopeless	0	1	2	3
3 Trouble falling or staying asleep, or sleeping too much	0	1	2	3
4 Feeling tired or having little energy	0	1	2	3
5 Poor appetite or overeating	0	1	2	3
6 Feeling bad about yourself or feeling that you are a failure or have let yourself or your family down	0	1	2	3
7 Trouble concentrating on things, such as reading the newspaper or watching television	0	1	2	3
8 Moving or speaking so slowly that other people could have noticed, or the opposite, being so fidgety or restless you have been moving around a lot more than usual	0	1	2	3
9 Thoughts that you would be better off dead or hurting yourself in some way	0	1	2	3

The PHQ 9 is now in public domain and freely available for use. See the website www.phqscreeners.com for more information.

Anxiety

Over the last 2 weeks, how often have you been bothered by any of the problems listed in Table A2.2? Please circle the number that best applies to you for each question.

Table A2.2 General Anxiety Disorder Scale (GAD-7) to measure levels of anxiety

GAD – 7	*Not at all*	*Several days*	*More than half the days*	*Nearly every day*
1 Feeling nervous, anxious or on edge	0	1	2	3
2 Not being able to stop or control worrying	0	1	2	3
3 Worrying too much about different things	0	1	2	3
4 Trouble relaxing	0	1	2	3
5 Being so restless that it is hard to sit still	0	1	2	3
6 Becoming easily annoyed or irritable	0	1	2	3
7 Feeling afraid as if something awful might happen	0	1	2	3

The GAD 7 is now in public domain and freely available for use. See the website www.phqscreeners.com for more information.

How to score the questionnaires

Chest pain frequency: This is a useful measure to take at baseline and to use throughout therapy, as well as at the end of treatment. If chest pain frequency reduces during treatment, this can be used to support the usefulness of your approach.

Chest pain severity: This is a simple measure of severity rated on a 0–10 scale. Again, severity at baseline can simply be compared to severity during or at the end of treatment to assess whether any changes have occurred during treatment.

Chest pain interference: This score can help to develop insight into how much chest pain is interfering with a person's life. It is calculated as the *average* of the three items asking about how distressing chest pain is, how much it interferes with everyday life and how much of a problem it is.

Negative beliefs about chest pain: This score can help to develop insight into the beliefs about chest pain at the start of treatment and whether these change over time. Each item is scored individually as the score given on the 0–10 scale.

Depression (PHQ-9): Calculate a total score based on all nine items. This can screen for the severity of depression. It can also demonstrate changes in depression over time. The screening scores for depression are: 0–4 = none; 5–9 = mild; 10–14 = moderate; 15–19 = moderately severe; 20–27 = severe depression. Any person scoring 10 or more can be regarded as suffering from clinically significant symptoms of depression.

Anxiety (GAD-7): Calculate a total score based on all seven items. This can screen for the severity of anxiety. It can also demonstrate changes in anxiety over time. The screening scores for anxiety are: 0–5 = mild; 6–10 = moderate; 11–15 = moderately severe; 16–21 = severe anxiety. Any person scoring eight or more can be regarded as suffering from clinically significant symptoms of anxiety.

Full Biopsychosocial Assessment Schedule

Spend time welcoming the patient to your specialist chest pain clinic, and put the patient at ease. Explain why they are here and who referred them. Reiterate that they were referred because of persistent chest pain and test results showing it is not related to the heart. This is a common experience, which is why there is a special clinic.

Check to see if they read the preassessment leaflet. Explain that chest pain can be caused by medical problems but just as often it is caused by other issues as well, including psychological and social factors, such as stress. This is why you have a whole hour now to find out more about their chest pain and their life more generally. The physician may do a brief physical exam. Before you begin on the structured assessment, collect the questionnaires and answer any pressing questions. (See Table A2.3.)

Table A2.3 Schedule for conducting a full biopsychosocial assessment

1	**General questions (psychologist): When did you first notice chest pain?** What happened at that time? What else was happening in your life at this time? Sometimes people find chest pain starts during or after a stressful time in their life. Do you think this applies to you? Had you ever had chest pain before this time?		
2	**Presenting problem (cardiologist): Can you describe the chest pain?** Does it occur during or after exercise? Does it make you stop or slow down? Does anything else cause the chest pain? What is the frequency and duration? What is the site and radiation? Does it vary in position? Does anything relieve the chest pain?		
3	**Guy's chest pain questionnaire**		
	Typicality score 0–3; 0=non-cardiac / 1–2=atypical / 3=typical	**Typical Score 1 if:**	**Atypical Score 0 if:**
	1 If you have 10 pains (or tightness or breathlessness) in a row, how many occur on exercise?	10	0–9
	2 How many occur at rest?	0–1	2–10
	3 How long does the pain last?	≤5 min	>5 min
4	**Impact (psychologist): How has chest pain affected your life as a whole?** Assess across domains of life including relationships, work, activity, family life.		

continued

Table A2.3 (Continued)

5 Chest pain cycle (psychologist): Can you tell me about a recent, typical chest pain episode?

Thoughts: What do you think is happening, before, during or after chest pain? What goes through your mind? Does this change if the pain is very bad? Do you worry that something bad will happen? What?
Prompts: You'll collapse, have a heart attack, die, embarrass yourself

Emotions: What you feel during chest pain? Did you notice any emotions? What do you feel like after chest pain?
Prompts: Scared, frustrated, sad, worried

Behaviour: What did/do you do during and after chest pain?
Is there anything that helps you to cope? Why do you think this helps?
Do you find yourself focusing on the pain, or do you try to ignore it?
Do you try to avoid chest pain? What and why do you do this? Does it work?
Prompt: Stop activities, avoid stress, rest, seek help, drink water

Body: Do you notice any other body sensations when you get chest pain?
Prompt: Breathless, feel hot or cold, sweaty, tingling, faint, dizzy, tense, aching

Social: How do other people respond to your chest pain? What do they do, say and think?
Since your chest pain began, have people treated you differently?
Prompt: Are they concerned? Do they encourage behaviours such as resting or help-seeking? Do they get upset or frustrated? Who is or is not supportive? What is this like for you?

Protective factors: What helps you to cope with your chest pain? What do you value in your life at the moment?

6 Personal and social history (cardiologist): Do you have any family history of chest pain?

If so, who? Do you have any family history of serious disease or heart disease? Does this affect the way you think about your own chest pain?

7 Psychiatric screening (psychologist): Other than chest pain, how are you feeling in yourself at the moment?

Depression: Check the PHQ-9 score (10 is clinical cut-off, 20 is a red flag).
How is your mood? Do you feel sad or tearful or hopeless? Have you noticed change in your sleep, appetite, or libido? Do you ever have thoughts or hurting yourself or taking your life?

Anxiety: Check GAD-7 score (10 is clinical cut-off, 15 is a red flag).
Do you ever get anxious? Do worry about things much of the time?

Panic: Do you get panic attacks? Do they happen with chest pain? What causes them?

Illness anxiety: Other than chest pain, do you tend to worry about your health?

Other: Have you ever been diagnosed with a mental health problem in the past? Do you ever struggle with intrusive thoughts or memories that distress you?

8 Stress (psychologist): Is there anything in your life at the moment that is very stressful that you haven't mentioned yet?

Work, relationships, conflict finances, housing, recent losses or changes
Have you noticed whether stress has an effect on your chest pain?

9 Other organic causes of chest pain (cardiologist)

Breathlessness
Air hunger
Breathlessness, especially during eating or talking
Sighing, gasping, throat clearing, globus
Pins and needles around the mouth or fingers (can be on left or right side)

Hyperacusis or photophobia (dark glasses with no opthalmological need)

Physical exam shows evidence of breathing abnormally:
Thoracic respiratory pattern
Localized tenderness
Breath holding time reduced (<20 seconds)
Voluntary overbreathing test for 30 seconds induces pain at rest
Gastrointestinal
Is there acid reflux, water brash, dysphagia?
Does the pain occur after food, with particular types of food or when lying or bending?
Is the pain relieved by antacids, fluids or eating?
Are there symptoms of irritable bowel (variable stool consistency, mucus, precipitancy, bloating, flatulence)?
Musculoskeletal
Do you have morning stiffness?
Does the pain happen with moving the neck or other joints?

Physical exam shows evidence of a musculoskeletal abnormality:
Springing of the spine
Movement of the neck
Crepitus and immobility at shoulder
Localized tenderness (Do you have to rub the area?)

10 Cardiac risk factors (cardiologist)
Do you smoke? How much?
Do you drink or use substances? How much?
Is there a family history of cardiac disease?
Assessment for hypertension, abnormal lipid levels and diabetes.

11 Review previous investigations and medications (cardiologist)

12 Goals for treatment (psychologist)
What would be your goals for treatment? Other than reducing chest pain, would you like anything else in your life to change?
If your chest pain were no longer so distressing or intrusive, what would you be doing differently? What would other people see you doing if you felt better?

Discussion

Allow the patient a chance to ask any questions. We found it helped to have a few minutes for the clinicians to discuss the assessment without the patient present, and we would ask them to wait in the waiting room as we did this. This time is used to compare clinical opinions and clarify the plan for treatment. If not yet done, there is also time to complete the patient's individual chest pain cycle.

Feedback

Bring the patient back to the room. Share their chest pain cycle and options for treatment. Answer any questions. Give the patient the information leaflet after assessment (handout 1 in Appendix 3) that summarizes the biopsychosocial model of chest pain and arrange further meetings.

Appendix 3

Treatment handouts

Initial handout

Handout 1: information following assessment and how to understand and manage chest pain

You have seen the cardiologist (heart specialist) and psychologist/nurse today in our clinic. **The cardiologist is confident that your heart is not the cause of your chest pain.** This leaflet explains more about what might be causing your pain and gives information about what can help.

What is causing my chest pain?

Chest pain that is unrelated to the heart is very common, and it affects up to 30% of people in the UK. Studies show that up to three-quarters of people attending specialist chest pain clinics have pain that is unrelated to the heart. Most people with chest pain have healthy hearts and their pain is caused by something else. Other common *biological* causes of chest pain include:

- Pain in the muscles between the ribs (caused by tension in these muscles).
- Pain in the chest wall (caused by strains or tears in the muscles or ligaments).
- Unhelpful breathing (breathing too fast or using the chest muscles too much).
- Digestive causes, such as spasm, tightening or inflammation of the oesophagus (the food pipe from the throat to the stomach) or ulcers.
- Pain coming from pinched nerves in the neck or back.

These causes are *not* medically serious. This means you can safely return to living your normal life without letting chest pain limit what you do.

Our cardiologist has checked you and reviewed your medical history. If any of the above causes are likely, this should have been discussed this with you, and you may even have been asked to see another specialist or begin a medication that may help.

What else can help?

We know that chest pain can have a major effect on someone's life. It can change how you think and feel, what you do and your relationships with other people. Chest pain is influenced not only by your body (biological factors) but also by your emotions and behaviours (psychological factors) and general life circumstances (social factors). This is called a *biopsychosocial* picture of chest pain. You have told us about what your chest pain makes you think, feel and do, and how other people react. We may also have found that you tend to have chest pain if you are thinking, feeling or acting in certain way.

Our clinic can help you to learn how to cope with chest pain when it happens and how to make changes in your life that could reduce the frequency of chest pain, and that should improve your general well-being. For example, you can learn breathing and relaxation techniques that will reduce muscle tension and strain in the chest; you can find ways to increase your activity and return to living life in a way that you want; you can learn how to manage issues in your life that may affect chest pain or cause stress. We will give you reliable, evidence-based information that we hope will make you feel less concerned about chest pain.

Is my chest pain dangerous?

No, your chest pain is not dangerous because it is not coming from your heart. Yet, many people with chest pain do think that chest pain is dangerous. Common thoughts include:

- Chest pain means that I have a serious heart problem.
- Chest pain is a sign of a heart attack.
- My chest pain means that I have angina.
- Chest pain is always dangerous, and if I have it then I might die.

None of these thoughts are true because *heart problems have been excluded for you.* Instead, your chest pain is caused by something else that is *not* serious and *not* life-threatening. Try to remind yourself that your chest pain is not a sign of danger, as this might help you feel better.

Avoiding a vicious cycle

The biological, psychological and social factors common in chest pain all affect one another. This forms a vicious cycle that keeps chest pain going and can even make it worse. This is shown in the following diagram. The most important factors will vary between people, so think about which parts of the cycle are most relevant to you.

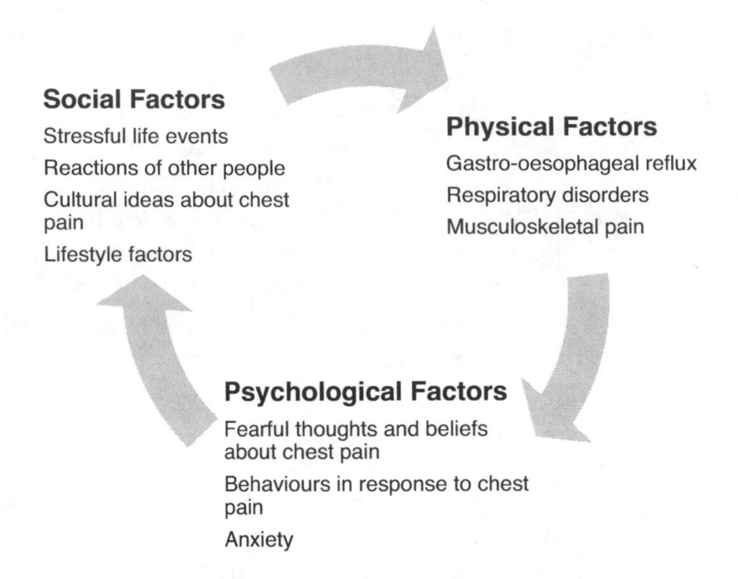

A biopsychosocial model of non-cardiac chest pain

What can help?

Changing beliefs and concerns about chest pain (and managing stress)

If you believe that your chest pain is dangerous, you will feel concerned about it. You may well have other stresses or worries in your life, too, such as at home or work, finances and so on. Concern and stress have an effect on the body, causing muscle tension, overbreathing and other physical symptoms. These changes from stress can cause chest pain. Learning to manage the physical symptoms of stress and learning to be less concerned about chest pain will help.

Changing what you do

You might have changed what you do because of chest pain, possibly becoming less active. Maybe this is because you think you need to protect your heart or feel that activity makes chest pain worse. However, avoiding activity makes chest pain worse over time. If you *keep active,* you will be fitter and healthier, feel better and be looking after your heart. If you can live a full and normal life, chest pain will be less of a problem. We can help you achieve this.

Emotions and mood

Chest pain can make you feel scared, fed-up, irritated, frustrated or sad. These feelings will be worse if you have stopped doing the things you enjoy or need to do and if you are worried about your health. We can help you to manage these emotions and find ways to help you improve your mood.

Focusing too much on chest pain

You probably now spend more time focusing on your body and chest than you used to do before you first got chest pain. When you pay attention to the body and to pain, it tends to make it feel worse and you become more aware of (even minor) changes in the body that you would previously have ignored. An example of the power of attention is the soldier injured in battle who reports not feeling pain because their attention is completely focused on survival. Since we can only pay attention to a few things at once, we feel less pain when we are distracted. Learning to distract your attention away from the chest pain onto something else can help.

Social factors

The way that other people react might affect how you think and feel about it. In our society, chest pain is regarded as a serious symptom, and this is true *only when* the heart is involved. Naturally, other people will worry and probably encourage you to seek help and keep resting. This is appropriate at first, but now that medical investigations have ruled out heart problems, this reaction can be unhelpful and make chest pain seem more dangerous than it is. Sometimes health care advice can be confusing and worrying, especially if you are told there is 'nothing wrong', despite your persistent chest pain. We aim to give clear advice based on the assessment where your heart was found to be healthy and to identify an alternative explanation so that you and other people in your life can feel less concerned.

An example of how these factors work in pain

Acute (new-onset) pain is our body's alarm system, warning us that there is an immediate health threat. However, pain that lasts for a long time (chronic pain) is different. Here, the alarm keeps going off without any immediate health threat. This can be very difficult to cope with. Pain is experienced in the brain and therefore involves *emotion* as well as *physical sensation*. The way that pain feels is affected by what it means to us. The meaning will depend on where the pain is coming from and your thoughts about it. If we think that pain is not threatening us, it will feel less severe than if we believe it threatens our existence or health. Similarly, the meaning of pain affects what we do, and if we think the pain threatens us, we do something to reduce the threat. The example in the table below shows how different ways of thinking about pain (headache and chest pain) change how we feel and what we do.

How the way we think about pain affects our experience of it

Type of pain	*Thoughts*	*Emotion*	*Action*	*Pain*
Headache	I am dehydrated and tired. Low threat	Neutral	Drink water and go to bed, pay little attention to pain.	Mild to moderate
Headache	I have a brain tumour. High threat	Fear	Worry, can't sleep and go to doctor, keep monitoring pain.	Severe
Chest pain	I have acid reflux. Low threat	Neutral/some annoyance	Drink a glass of water/take an antacid, ignore pain.	Moderate
Chest pain	I have heart disease. High threat	Anxiety	Worry, rest, go to A&E, focus on pain.	Severe

The types of thoughts you have about your own pain will be personal and will depend on all the other things happening in your life now and in the past. In our clinic, we will work with you to better understand your chest pain, so that you can learn to manage it more effectively.

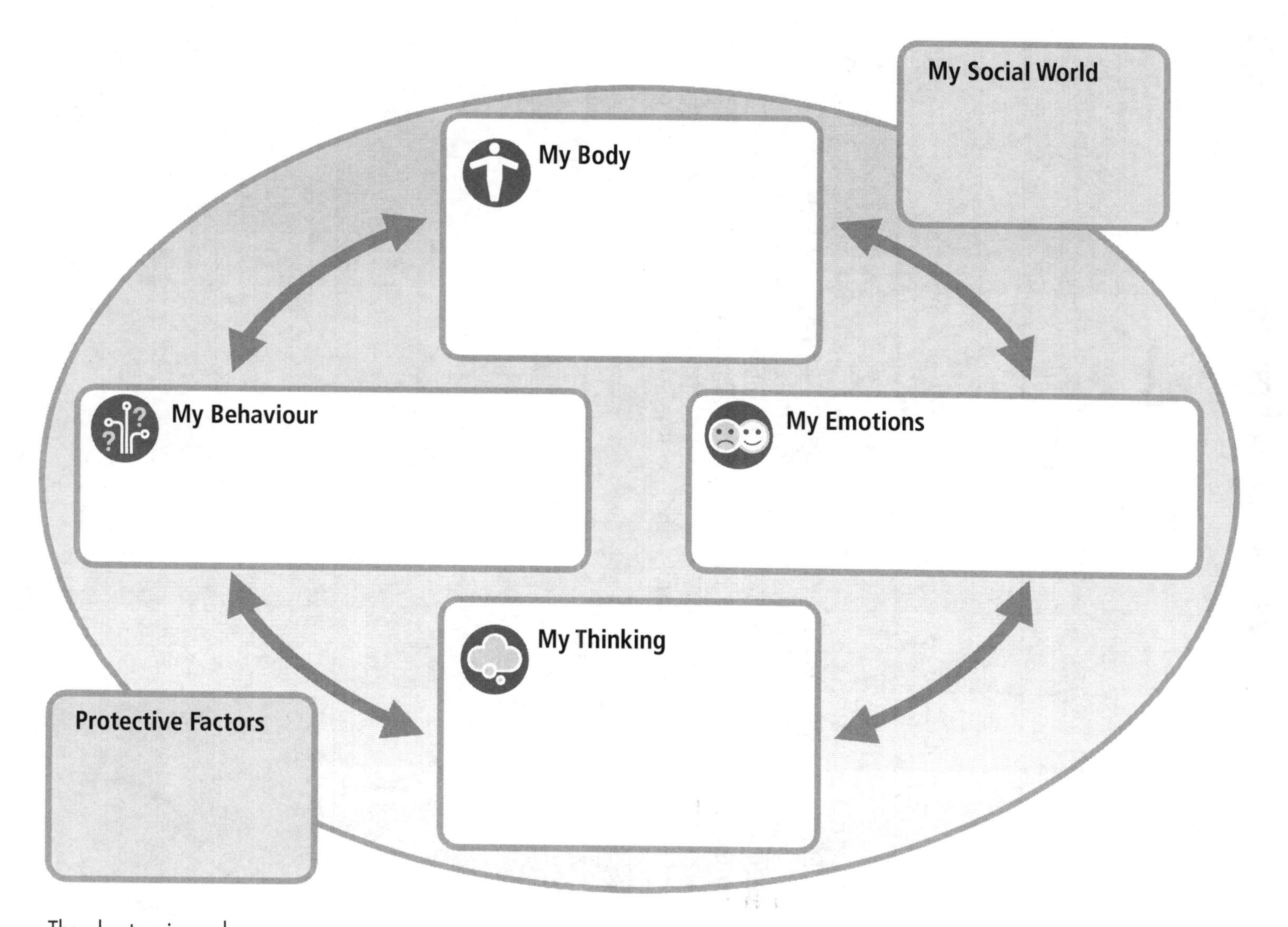

The chest pain cycle

HANDOUTS FOR SESSION 1

Handout 2: Goals for treatment

We have talked about how chest pain has affected your life and what you want to change. It is helpful to set some goals that you would like to reach by coming to these sessions. Try to think of SMART goals:

Specific Measurable Achievable Realistic Time-Limited

What do you want to be different by the end of treatment? Think about what you would be doing if things changed for the better or what other people might notice. How will we know if you've reached your goals by the time we finish our work together? For goals that might take longer to reach, what smaller, interim goals might you need to reach first?

Rather than having no pain at all, it might be more realistic to focus on what you can do, such as exercising again, first by walking for 10 minutes three times a week and building up to every day. Another goal could be to worry less about the pain and to start to enjoy life again. This could be measured by your activity and also by how you feel day to day.

My goals for treatment

1

2

3

4

5

Handout 3: Homework following session 1

- You can review the clinic information leaflet, your chest pain cycle and your goals, and think about what we have discussed today.
- If you think of any new goals, write these down, too.
- Keep a chest pain diary over the next week.

Handout 4: Chest pain dairy

Instructions for the chest pain diary

Sometimes chest pain is triggered by certain situations or activities. This may or may not be obvious, so keeping a diary can help us look for patterns and chest pain triggers.

Whenever you have chest pain over the next week, write it in your diary. Try to include what happens before, during and after the pain.

- *Before and during the pain:* What exactly happened? When was it? Where were you? What were you doing? Who else was there?
- *Chest pain:* What did it feel like? How bad was it (on a scale of 0–10)? Did you feel anything else in your body?
- *Emotions:* What emotions did you feel (scared, worried, sad, frustrated, irritated)?
- *Thinking:* What went through your mind when you had chest pain? Did you focus on the pain or on something else?
- *Behaviour:* What did you do when you noticed the chest pain? What did other people do?

An example of what to write is in the first row of the diary.

The chest pain diary

Use as many sheets as you need, and whenever you have an episode of chest pain, make a note of what happens. An example has been provided for you in the first row.

Situation	*Chest pain and severity*	*Emotions*	*Thoughts*	*Behaviours*
When was it? Where were you? What were you doing? Who was there?	What was the pain like? severity (0–10)	What emotions did you feel (e.g. scared, sad, worried, irritated)?	What went through your mind? What did you think was happening?	What did you do? What did other people do?
EXAMPLE: At work, Tuesday afternoon, talking to a client on phone	*Stabbing chest pain 8 = bad*	*Stressed, overwhelmed*	*I'm going to lose that client. I'm having a heart attack.*	*I told my boss and she told me to go home and rest.*

HANDOUTS FOR SESSION 2

Handout 5: Helpful breathing

Ways of breathing

There are two different ways to breathe. One way mainly uses the chest, so it is called *chest breathing*. The other way mainly moves the abdomen, so it is called *abdominal breathing*. Chest breathing is often used when we are stressed, excited or are doing extreme exercise. You may notice this yourself, as the chest moves up and down a lot. Sometimes people develop a habit of using chest breathing most of the time. This is often associated with intermittent gasping or throat-clearing. Chest breathing can cause unpleasant sensations, including chest pain. Family or friends may notice this more than you.

Chest (unhelpful) breathing

Chest breathing happens when we draw air into the chest. The chest and shoulders move up and down with each breath, and air only enters the top of our lungs so our lungs don't expand fully. Your breaths are probably *fast*, *irregular*, *shallow* or *gasping*. This sort of chest breathing is unhelpful because it can cause unpleasant sensations such as:

- Breathlessness at rest, with minimal activity, or when talking or eating
- Feeling suffocated or unable to take a satisfying breath
- Feeling restricted, trapped or confined
- Fatigue, often for prolonged periods after exertion
- Dizziness or muzzy head
- Pins and needles in the fingers or around the mouth
- Headaches
- Blurred vision or bright light hurts the eyes
- Startle easily with loud noises
- Muscle tension and pain in the shoulders
- Tight chest, heaviness or pressure (may need to loosen clothing around the chest)
- Chest pain
- Palpitations (fast heartbeat or overawareness of normal heart beat).

Abdominal (helpful) breathing

It is possible to learn to use a more helpful breathing style, where the movement of the breath is in the diaphragm and the abdomen. This type of breathing will reduce muscle tension and stress around the chest, which are common causes of causes of chest pain.

Understanding the breath

Our lungs fill a cavity in our chest composed of the ribs at the sides and the diaphragm at the bottom. The diaphragm is a dome-shaped muscle at the bottom of the lungs that is very flexible. To take a breath in, we must increase the size of the chest cavity, usually by contracting the diaphragm so that it becomes flat. As the cavity size increases, air is drawn into the lungs.

Why abdominal breathing is more helpful

The chest wall has limited flexibility, and the muscles between the ribs are small and weak. Moving the chest up and down causes strain on the chest muscles without actually increasing the size of the cavity very much. On the other hand, the diaphragm is very flexible and strong and does not become strained during breathing. It also increases the size of the cavity significantly.

How do I usually breathe?

To find out, put one hand on your stomach and the other on your chest. Take a slow, deep breath in. If your ribs, shoulders or chest move up or out and your stomach doesn't move, then you are using chest breathing.

Learning abdominal breathing

To breathe in, remember that the chest does not have to move. Instead, imagine that the breath travels all the way down into the abdomen (stomach area). As the diaphragm contracts it is flattened, and it will push down on the stomach. This will make the stomach area rise.

To breathe out, the diaphragm relaxes and returns to its dome shape. This allows the stomach to flatten once more. The chest cavity decreases in size and the air is pushed out as the lungs empty. In abdominal breathing, your chest should stay still whilst your stomach moves in and out. The following diagram shows you how this works.

Try it for yourself. It is often easiest to begin to learn this way of breathing when you are lying down, either flat or with your knees bent. Place one hand on your stomach and the other on your chest. Try to breathe slowly just with the stomach. Keep your stomach muscles relaxed so that your stomach rises when you breathe in. When you breathe out, let

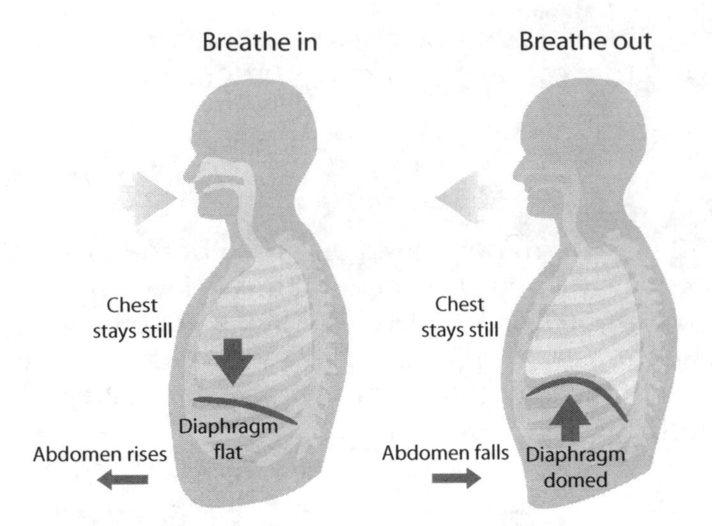

Diagram demonstrating abdominal breathing styles

your stomach sink back down. Try to keep your chest still throughout. Aim for about 8–12 breaths per minute, trying not to gasp, hold your breath, sigh or clear your throat.

Handout 6: Homework following session 2

Learning abdominal breathing

This skill takes time and practice to learn. Try the following homework exercises:

- Set aside a regular time to practise abdominal breathing for 10 minutes each day. Use the CD to guide you. Lie (or sit) somewhere comfortable.
- Several times a day, pause and breathe. Throughout the day, stop for a moment and take a few slow abdominal breaths. Use a reminder, like an hourly alarm on your phone or watch, or put stickers or notes somewhere obvious to you. Write down what you will use here,

To remind myself to use abdominal breathing throughout the day, I will:

- Breathe in response to difficulty and chest pain. When you feel confident using abdominal breathing, it can be a useful way of coping with stress and chest pain. When stress and pain arise, choose to focus on your breathing. Begin to take slow, paced abdominal breaths (not too deeply) and notice what happens.
- See what difference abdominal breathing makes to you by recording what happens when you do the exercises using the following breathing diary.

The breathing diary

Over the next 1 or 2 weeks, make a note of when you use abdominal breathing and the effect this has on how you feel. An example has been provided for you in the first row.

Situation (day, time, what is happening)	*How I felt in this situation (e.g. stress, panic, chest pain, hot, tense)*	*How I felt after doing abdominal breathing (chest pain, tension, stress and breathing, anything else)*
Example: Tuesday 2 p.m., difficult phone call at work	*Very stressed, strong pain in chest, tense shoulders*	*Less stressed, less shoulder tension and chest pain*
Situation 1		
Situation 2		
Situation 3		
Situation 4		
Situation 5		
Situation 6		
Situation 7		

HANDOUTS FOR SESSION 3

Handout 7: Stress, anxiety and chest pain

Stress and anxiety are normal reactions to threat. Feeling under threat will cause the body to release hormones which lead to changes in the body and mind that prepare us to cope with potential danger. The body is made ready to fight or run from a threat, so we call this the *fight or flight response*. Changes are seen in breathing (which gets faster and tends to involve the chest more), the heart (which beats faster, pumping blood to the muscles), and the muscles (which get tense and ready for action). We might sweat (to cool the body), and our senses (sight and hearing) sharpen. The mind will focus more on looking out for possible threat (see the following figure). These changes are normal and adaptive, because this reaction enabled our species to survive environmental challenges (such as fighting or escaping a dangerous predator, such as a tiger).

Threats in modern life are different and aren't always solved by fight or flight, for example, stressful situations involving big demands

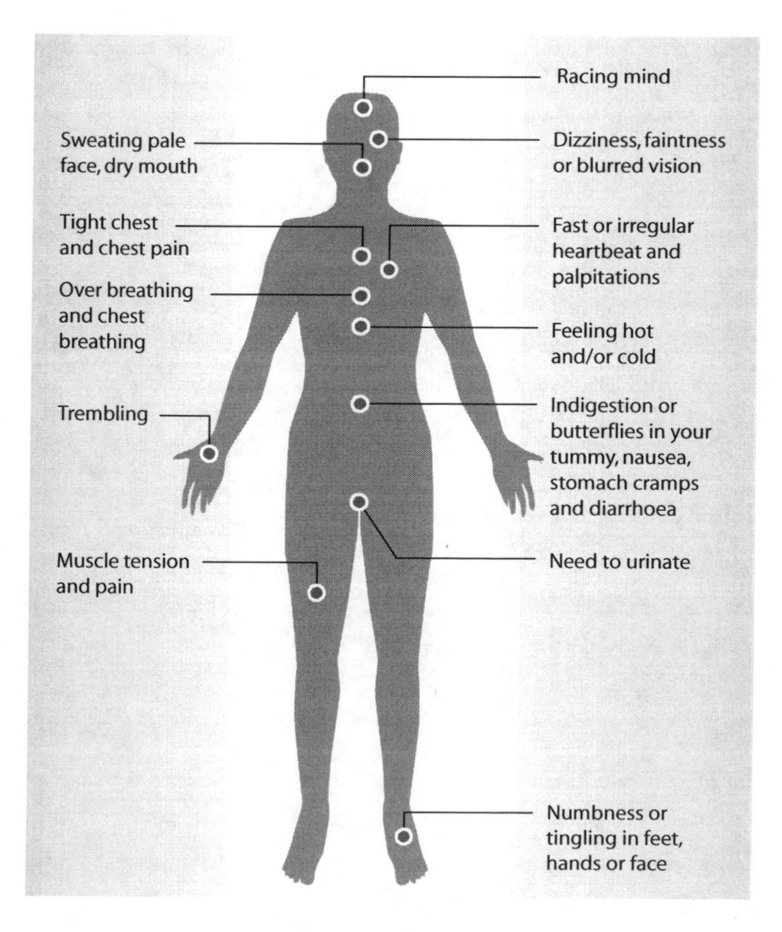

Physical sensations and physiological changes that can occur with stress

or difficult problems (with work, money, relationships or health). The brain reacts to these chronic stressors in the same way as that it reacts to acute threats (like tigers!). So chronic stress triggers a flight or flight response, even if this is not going to solve the problem. This means that long-term stressors can lead to an on-going stress response.

Some of the most common physical symptoms that arise with stress and anxiety are chest sensations. This is due to

- Muscle tension arising in the chest wall
- Increased breathing rate (and reliance on chest breathing)
- Increased heart rate and palpitations.

These body sensations are *not dangerous*. They are just part of anxiety. However, if you are worried about them, it can feed your chest pain cycle.

My own vicious cycle of stress

Think of a time in the last few weeks when you can remember yourself feeling stressed, scared or under pressure. When was this, where were you and what was happening?

What emotions were you feeling?

What was happening in your body?

Do you remember what you were thinking?

Do you remember what you were paying most attention to?

Handout 8: Problem solving

- Focus on one problem at a time. What do you want to achieve?
- Start with an easier problem to give you a chance to learn this technique before trying to solve more difficult or complicated problems.
- Identify which problems are *important* and then solve them.

The problem-solving table

Identify What is the specific problem? What do you want to achieve? Break down complex problems into smaller, easier parts.	
Brainstorm Write down *any* and *all* possible solutions. Have an open mind, and don't judge any solution at this stage. No matter how silly a solution is, write it down.	
Consequences Write down the pros and cons of each solution. What are the consequences of each?	
Choose one What is the best possible solution?	
Plan it Make a careful plan about how to try this solution. What will you do? How will you do it? When? Where? Will anyone help you? Are there potential problems? Can you avoid them?	
Do it Carefully follow your plan.	
Evaluate it What happened? Did you progress at all? Were there any problems with the plan?	
If you solved your problem, what do you need to do now to keep the problem solved? If you solved just one part of a larger problem, repeat this exercise with the other parts.	
If your problem is not solved, can you change your plan so it is more effective? Can you try another solution from your list?	

Handout 9: Homework following session 3

Practise relaxation regularly

Chest pain is often caused by muscle tension around the ribs, shoulders and back. Sometimes chest pain is made worse by stress or anxiety. Relaxation works on the body to reduce muscle tension and they physical changes of stress. It can help you manage chest pain.

- Practise relaxation for 20 minutes every day, using track 5 on the audio guide.
- Fill in the relaxation diary to see what happens to stress, tension and chest pain when you relax.
- After a few weeks, start using shorter relaxation exercises (track 6 on the audio guide).
- Continue to do 10 minutes of breathing exercises each day, and regularly check in with your breathing.
- If discussed in the session, follow your problem-solving plan to reduce stress.

Tips for practising relaxation

- Try to find a warm, quiet place where you can be alone and undisturbed for 20 minutes. Silence your phone and ask people not to interrupt you.
- Choose a position where you are safe if you fall asleep (sitting on a comfortable chair or lying down). *Do not* listen to the relaxation audio guides while driving or using tools or machinery.

Common difficulties

- Your mind will wander away from the guided exercise. It may feel frustrating, but this is normal. Just notice where your mind has gone and then gently refocus on the exercise or your breathing.
- You might fall asleep. This is not a problem, but it may make it harder to learn the relaxation exercises. Try sitting up and keeping your eyes open.
- The feeling of relaxation may feel strange or uncomfortable. This is normal and feels easier with time. You may prefer to open your eyes.

Applying relaxation to your daily life

You can bring relaxation into your daily life in the same way you did abdominal breathing. Throughout the day, check in with your body and do the following:

1 Adjust your *posture* to be upright but relaxed.
2 *Scan* through your body, and if you feel tension, let it relax.
3 Drop your shoulders and let your jaw relax.
4 *Take a slow breath* in, and then relax as you breathe out.
5 If you have chest pain, see what happens if you just allow it to be there. Don't fight it, but instead focus your attention on the breath in your abdomen and breathe slowly and gently until it passes.

Relaxation diary

Over the next 1 or 2 weeks, make a note of when you use relaxation exercises and the effect these have on how you feel. An example has been provided for you in the first row, and we will complete another example when we practise relaxation in our session.

Situation **When I plan to practise each day.**	**How I feel before relaxation. Rate tension, stress and chest pain.** **0 = none to 10 = severe**	**How I feel after relaxation. Rate tension, stress and chest pain.** **0 = none to 10 = severe**
Example: *Day 1: Wednesday, 7 p.m., before dinner, in lounge, worrying about work tomorrow*	Tension = 9 (all body) Stressed = 7 Chest pain = 2	Tension = 3 (better) Stress = 4 (better) Chest pain = 2 (same)
Practise in session at the chest pain clinic	**Tension in body =** **Stress =** **Chest pain =**	**Tension in body =** **Stress =** **Chest pain =**
Day 1		
Day 2		
Day 3		
Day 4		
Day 5		
Day 6		
Day 7		

HANDOUTS FOR SESSION 4

Handout 10: Activity and chest pain – the facts

Many people with persistent chest pain become less active over time. They might stop doing things that are important or fun. They often exercise less. Sometimes this is because activity triggers chest pain. Sometimes they even worry that exercise will harm them, but *this is not the case!*

Medical advice for people with or without chest pain is similar: gradually increase your activity and exercise at a level that raises your heart rate.

Regular, moderate activity improves health and well-being

- It makes your body and heart fitter and stronger.
- It lowers your blood pressure.
- It reduces your risk of heart disease.
- It improves immune function (the body's ability to protect against disease).
- It reduces stress and improves your mood.

Avoiding activity will make chest pain worse

Avoiding activity means your body loses strength and fitness. This can make chest pain worse because

- If muscles lose strength, they are more likely to be strained during activity.
- If the body loses fitness, you will be more breathless during activity.
- If you stop doing fun or important activities, you will probably feel more stressed and down and less independent.

Safety behaviours and avoidance are not helpful

People who avoid activity because of chest pain tend to become more fearful about chest pain and activity. When we avoid something we fear, we begin by feeling that we are staying safe. However, it also means we never get a chance to find out if our fears are true. Your doctors recommend keeping active, but you can only find out if this advice is right for you by experimenting and testing out what happens if you start doing activity again. If you have been inactive for a while, it is important to increase activity *slowly and gradually.*

Choose activities that fit with your goals for treatment and that are important to you. Consider how and why chest pain affects your life as you answer the following questions. Perhaps the chest pain cycle can help you.

How can I keep active?

1 If I woke up tomorrow with no chest pain, what would I start *doing?*
2 What do I value most in my life? (family, friends, other relationships, work, play, health, etc.)
3 What activities support the things I value and are enjoyable and important to me?
4 What were my original goals at the start of my treatment?
5 What activities am I *already doing now* that fit with my values and goals? How can I manage these, and how can I build on them?
6 What activities am I not doing or avoiding now because of chest pain?
7 Why am I no longer doing these things? What worries or concerns have stopped me?

Handout 11: Activity ladder

Based on your values and goals, choose what activities you want to start doing again. Rate the activity in terms of how difficult it is on a scale of 0–10. An activity rated as 0 involves no difficulty at all, and an activity rated as 10 is almost impossible.

Then write them in the following table *in order of difficulty,* with the easiest first.

The activity ladder

Difficulty rating (0–10)	**Activity (Be specific and include detail if you have decided to make it easier e.g. time doing activity, who with, where, how many rests).**

How to use the activity ladder

1. For the easiest activity, plan when and where you will do it over the next week in your diary. Plan in how you will seek support from other people if necessary.
2. Use your diary to record what you do and how doing an activity feels.
3. Be kind to yourself. Everyone finds it difficult to make changes. Don't push yourself too hard, and try to be realistic about what you can manage.
4. Reward yourself when you do an activity to help you stay motivated. Choose a reward that will make you feel good (e.g. do something fun, buy a small treat or tell others so they can praise you).

   What will *your* rewards be?

   ____

   ____

5. Be flexible. Unexpected things may occur (you may catch a cold or have a crisis at work), so you may need to change your plan to do something more manageable.
6. Involve family or friends who will support you when necessary.
7. Include pleasant activities, even small things, particularly if you have stopped doing them.
8. Move on gradually and only when your current activity has become easy (and you rate it as no more than a 1/10). It may take weeks or months before you can do the most difficult activity.

Beware the overactivity/resting cycle! If you try to increase your activity too quickly, it can make things worse. If you push yourself too much at first, you may get too tired; then you will have to rest and your body will lose even more strength and fitness. Take it slow.

Handout 12: Pacing and the overactivity/resting cycle

Long-term improvements depend on gradual increases in activity. Otherwise you might fall into the unhelpful overactivity/resting cycle:

- *Overactive!* On a good day, you might get a burst of energy and feel ready for anything. When you feel like this, it is tempting to do lots of activity, even more than planned. This can feel good at the time, but overexerting yourself in this way can have consequences the next day.
- *Rest!* After overexerting yourself, the body may be tired and need to rest. You may then do *less* activity than planned, or no activity at all, for several days.

If this happens repeatedly, the body will lose strength and fitness, and the next activity may feel even more difficult.

Pacing prevents this cycle. Pacing means that you follow a consistent activity plan every day, regardless of how you feel. You begin with the easiest activity you can manage (the baseline) and increase gradually as it becomes easier (probably about a 10% increase per week). Pacing can be frustrating, but it will help you improve quicker. Pacing can also be used during an activity by planning in regular rest breaks; for example, walk for 5 minutes, rest for 2 minutes and walk for another 5 minutes.

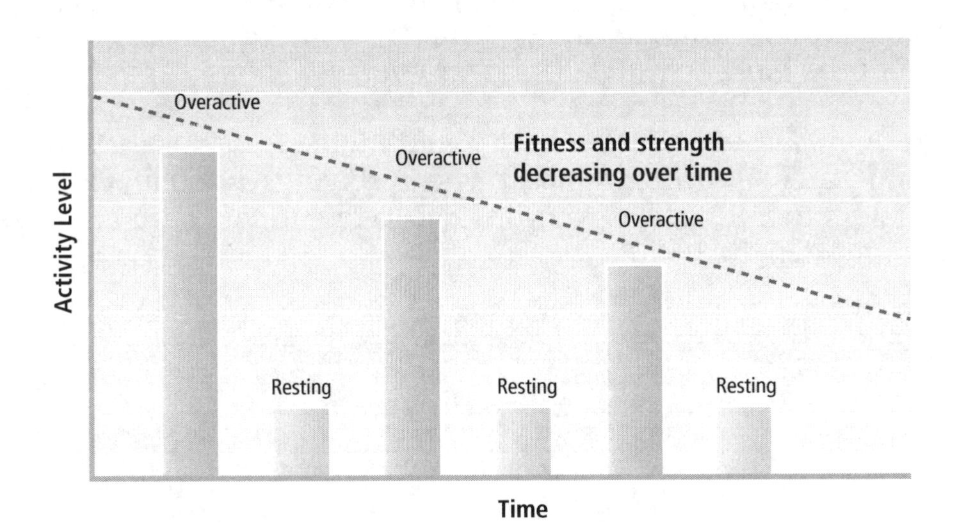

Diagram of overactivity/resting cycle

Handout 13: Homework following session 4

Keeping active

- Begin to work up your activity ladder, starting with the easiest activity.
- Plan when and where you will do this activity between now and our next session. Write this in your activity diary.
- Each time you do an activity, note what happens in your diary. If you can't manage an activity, write down why.

Pacing

- For the first week, don't go beyond your plan. The best results will come if you work up your activity ladder slowly. When your easiest activity has reduced to a 1/10 difficulty, you can move on to the next activity on your ladder.
- If you overdo it, don't worry. Try to keep going as planned.
- You can use pacing during an activity, too, by planning in regular rest breaks. Make sure you *plan these in advance,* rather than just stopping when you feel tired or in response to chest pain.

Keep going with your other strategies

- Practise relaxation and breathing regularly and try using these strategies when stress and chest pain arise.
- Continue with any problem-solving tasks if you discussed these today.

The activity diary

Try to complete a plan for increasing activity gradually over the next week by scheduling activities that you will do. Try to be specific about what you will do. An example is given in the first row.

Day	**Time (Plan an exact time)**	**Planned action/goal What you plan to do, where, how long, with whom; plan breaks (Remember to start with something easy)**	**Achieved? ☺ What helped? What made it difficult?**
Example: Saturday	*12 noon*	*Easiest activity on my ladder (4/10 difficulty): Walk for 15 minutes with my friend. Stop every 5 minutes for a 1-minute rest before continuing.*	*Achieved. No chest pain. Used breathing each rest. My friend helped me keep going. It was easier than expected, 3/10.*
1			
2			
3			
4			
5			

HANDOUTS FOR SESSION 5

Handout 14: Common beliefs about chest pain

Following is a list of some of the most common beliefs that people with chest pain have. Some of these beliefs are false, and some are true. First cover up the answers and then write down whether you think each belief is true or false.

Common beliefs about chest pain

As you compare your answers to the ones medical fact, what do you notice? Were you surprised to find out that any of the beliefs about chest pain were true or false?

Common belief about chest pain	**Your view: is it true or false?**	**Medical evidence: is it true or false?**
Chest pain is always a sign of an impending cardiac event.		False
Heart disease is directly caused by stress.		False
Chest pain can be caused by stress.		True
Rest is the best treatment for chest pain.		False
A raised heart rate will cause a heart attack.		False
If you have chest pain you will definitely have a heart attack.		False
If you have chest pain, you can live a normal, active life.		True
If I have chest pain, I must immediately control it or something terrible will happen.		False

Handout 15: Thinking more helpfully about chest pain

Worrying thoughts: Following are some common worries people have about chest pain. Circle any thoughts you have about chest pain, and write any others down, too.

Helpful thoughts: There are also some helpful thoughts offered as alternatives to these worries. Circle any of these which might apply to you. It may help to think about what you have learnt from treatment here, such as from your chest pain cycle, stress management strategies and activity plans. Add any other helpful thoughts of your own, too.

My chest pain means that I am:

Worrying thought: Having a heart attack/having angina/about to die
Helpful thought: Stressed/chest breathing/have indigestion/have muscle tension

My chest pain is caused by:

Worrying thought: Heart disease/a serious illness
Helpful thought: Less serious issues like stress/worry/acid reflux/overbreathing

The consequences of chest pain are:

Worrying thought: I will die/I will collapse/I won't be able to cope
Helpful thought: I might feel uncomfortable, but it will pass and I will then be okay.

Control over chest pain:

Worrying thought: I have no control over my chest pain.
Helpful thought: I have some control over my chest pain and I can cope if I use breathing/relaxation/distraction/something else: ______________

Any other thoughts you have:

Worrying thought:
More helpful thought:
Worrying thought:
More helpful thought:

Building up the alternative, helpful thoughts

1 **Rating your negative thoughts**
From the previous list, rate how much you believe each of the more helpful thoughts (on a scale of 0–10, where 0 means you don't believe the thought at all and 10 means you believe it completely).

2 **Understand your ratings**
If there are any helpful thoughts that you believe less than 7/10, can you think of what is stopping you from believing this thought more?

3 **Increase your ratings**
What have you learnt from treatment that might increase your belief rating?

What did your test results show?

What did the doctors say causes your chest pain?

What often triggers your chest pain? Why do we think this is?

What usually helps your chest pain? Why do we think this helps?

Have your fears about what chest pain might lead to ever happened?

If not, why do you think this is the case?

Over the past few weeks, what evidence have you gathered that suggests that your worrying thoughts may be false and that the more helpful thoughts may be true? For example, what have you learnt about how stress, breathing style, relaxation and activity affect your chest pain?

Handout 16: Helpful thoughts flashcard

Following is a list of helpful thoughts and beliefs about chest pain. These are based on experience and knowledge from working with chest pain, and they should fit with evidence you have collected over the past few weeks of treatment. There are blank spaces on the flashcard for you to fill in.

It is possible to make this more helpful way of thinking about chest pain more automatic. The best way to do this is to rehearse the thoughts in your mind regularly. Try the following:

1 Read your helpful thoughts flashcard regularly every day (e.g. when you get up or go to bed).
2 Try reading the sentences out loud to yourself.
3 Show the flashcard to someone else who might be able to help remind you or who worries about your chest pain so they can learn what you have learnt.
4 Put the flashcard up somewhere prominent you will see it every day.
5 Keep the flashcard with you wherever you go; make other copies and keep one in your bag or pocket.
6 Whenever you have chest pain or are worrying about it, read the flashcard and try to remember how you know these thoughts are true.

The flashcard will remind you of what you have learnt during treatment and may help you feel calmer and decide what to do that will help. Over time, these thoughts will become more habitual, and you may find that you no longer think so negatively about chest pain.

At times of pain or stress, it is harder to remember this way of thinking. For this reason, even if you already find these thoughts easy to believe, it is still worth keeping the flashcard and rehearing the thoughts regularly.

Helpful thoughts flashcard

Facts I know about my chest pain:

The doctor has checked my heart and is *confident that it is healthy.*
My chest pain is *not* caused by a serious heart condition or illness.
My chest pain is *not* a sign that I am about to have a heart attack.
My chest pain is *not* a sign of imminent danger.

My chest pain happens for less serious reasons, including: ______________________________

____

It is safe to carry on doing my normal activities when I have chest pain. I have done this before, for example: ______________________________
I can cope with chest pain and can have some control over it. For example, I can use skills such as: ______________________________________

____

Other things that help me to remember I'm okay despite chest pain are: ______________________

____

____

Handout 17: Attention and chest pain

When we are concerned about something, we tend to focus more on it. This can help when we need to be alert to danger (such as when crossing a road). However, it can be more problematic when we spend a lot of time focusing on something like our body. This is because when we pay attention to something, we notice more about it.

Selective attention and pain

The body has many different, changing sensations. This is normal, so we usually ignore them. However, if we are worried about our body or health, we probably pay more attention to sensations. This makes us more aware of what is happening in the body, which might make us anxious. Anxiety itself can then cause more physical sensations (including chest pain). This can feed into the chest pain cycle.

Refocusing attention

When you notice yourself monitoring your body sensations, remind yourself that this is unhelpful. Then choose to refocus your attention elsewhere. Choose an activity or mental exercise that is interesting or challenging enough to engage your mind, such as reading, listening to music, singing, thinking about a pleasant memory, imagining an interesting place, doing a crossword, playing Sudoku, playing a game on your phone, doing mental arithmetic, phoning a friend and so on. Choose a few options that will be available in different situations; for example, you might sing when you are alone, but you prefer to do a puzzle in public. Note your plan for refocusing attention.

My plan for refocusing attention to cope with stress or when I find myself monitoring my body sensations

Situation	**Refocusing attention activity**
Example: On the bus, I notice unusual sensations in my chest.	*Example: Do a crossword (I will carry a crosswords book in my bag).*

Handout 18: Homework following session 5

- *Use the helpful thoughts flashcard.* Follow the instructions on the helpful thoughts flashcard, and remember to use it every day (rehearsal) and when you have chest pain (response).
- *Attention and distraction.* If you have covered this in today's session, try to use your distraction activities whenever you notice yourself focusing on your chest area or when chest pain is happening. If not, you may like to read through handout 17 to learn more about this technique.
- *Continue with your activity plan.* Move onto the next stage on your ladder if you are ready. If not, note what your activity plan is for next week.

  ____

  ____

- *Continue with breathing and relaxation.* Do these regularly and in response to chest pain. If you have a strong preference for one technique, you can focus more on this. You can try the shorter version of relaxation (track 6) if you have not already done so; this is relaxation only (without tension), so can be done more easily when in public.

HANDOUT FOR SESSION 6

Handout 19: Review of progress and plan for maintaining positive changes

What have I noticed about my progress in coping with and managing my chest pain?

How have I changed the way that I think, feel and behave in response to chest pain?

How close have I come to meeting my goals for treatment?

What parts of treatment did I find most helpful, and what was less helpful? How did I use these strategies and what have they done to help me?

- Understanding what causes my chest pain and that it is not my heart
- Understanding thoughts, emotions, behaviours and the vicious chest pain cycle
- Learning abdominal, paced breathing
- Understanding stress and learning relaxation skills
- Using problem solving
- Testing out and increasing my activity in a graded and paced way
- Learning how to think more helpfully about chest pain

Identifying future goals

What are my future goals? Am I happy to maintain the changes I have already made? Or do I want to make more changes in my life that chest pain used to prevent?

Planning for the future

How will I work towards my goals? How do I plan to keep using helpful strategies in the future, whether to maintain the positive changes I have already made or move towards new goals?

Planning for future goals

	Goal	**Goal**	**Goal**	**Goal**
What do I plan to do?				
When do I plan to do it?				
Where do I plan to do it?				
How often do I plan to do it?				

Possible setbacks

What might lead to a setback? What might be a barrier to maintaining or making changes (lack of time, life stressors, interruptions, motivation, illness etc.)?

Indicators of setbacks

How will I know that I might be having a setback? Apart from chest pain, what might I or other people notice in what I do, say, think or feel that might indicate a setback?

Managing setbacks

If I do experience a setback, what can I do about it? What technique could I use that I have already learnt in treatment? Where can I seek appropriate support or help?

How can I minimize the risk of setbacks?

What should I keep doing to make a setback less likely? How can I keep going with helpful techniques and remind myself regularly (e.g. set aside an hour per month to read through my notes and remember what is useful)?

For the future

Try setting aside an hour each month for yourself, taking time to review your therapy notes, reflect on progress and plan what you can do next.

Glossary of terms

Angina – A sensation of pain or pressure in the chest caused by a reduced oxygen supply to the heart muscle. This is usually caused by coronary artery disease, less commonly by aortic stenosis and occasionally by thickening of the heart muscle as a result of hypertrophic cardiomyopathy. It is typically precipitated by exertion and relieved by rest.

Atheroma – Accumulation of cholesterol associated with inflammation, fibrosis and smooth muscle proliferation that leads to a reduction in the size of the lumen (see later) of an artery.

Behavioural experiment – Experiential activities conducted by the patient inside or outside of therapy to test out the validity of a belief or theory.

Biopsychosocial model – A broad perspective that accounts for multiple factors (biological, psychological and social) in the causes, maintenance and outcomes of disease and illness.

Catastrophizing – A style of negative thinking which involves imagining the worst-case scenario associated with a particular experience or event. It is often associated with worrying.

CBT (cognitive behavioural therapy) – A psychotherapy designed to help alleviate distress associated with physical and mental health problems by changing unhelpful patterns of thinking and behaviour.

Cervical spondylosis – Degenerative changes in the bones of the neck that lead to stiffness and pain in the neck that can also radiate to the head or upper chest.

Cognitions – A person's thoughts, beliefs and interpretations about themselves, other people, the world or any other experience.

Cognitive restructuring – Learning to identify negative thinking patterns and changing these to more helpful thinking patterns using various CBT techniques.

Computerised tomography – An imaging procedure based on X-ray that can create detailed scans of the interior of the body.

Electrocardiogram (ECG) – A test that measures the electrical activity of the heart.

Fibromyalgia – A chronic condition characterized by musculoskeletal and joint pain and particular points of localized tenderness in the body.

Formulation – The shared understanding between a therapist and a patient about all of the factors involved in a patient's experience of chest pain. This will include the physical sensations, thoughts, emotions, behaviours and social context that are associated with chest pain.

Gate control theory – A theoretical understanding of pain which accounts for both the physical and psychological aspects of pain perception.

Hypervigilance – An increased sensitivity to one's environment with an intent to detect threat. This is usually associated with anxiety and behavioural changes, as well as selective attention.

Hypocapnia – A state of reduced carbon dioxide in the blood caused by hyperventilation which may lead to changes in arterial blood flow or nerve function.

Lumen – The inside space of a blood vessel.

Mindfulness – A meditation technique that often involves a focus on the breath or body and learning to remain in the present moment, which can lead to reduction in stress and improvements in psychological well-being.

Myocardial infarction (i.e. heart attack or coronary thrombosis) – Occurs when blockage of a coronary artery leads to damage to the heart muscle supplied by that artery.

Myocardial ischaemia – Restriction of blood supply to the heart usually leading to chest pain or breathlessness on exercise (angina) and sometimes to abnormal rhythms or progressive damage to the heart muscle.

Normalizing – A form of education where evidence is given that the patient's experiences are commonly reported by other people (e.g. that NCCP is prevalent and usually benign).

Oesophageal motility disorder – Uncoordinated, prolonged or abnormally high pressure contractions of the smooth muscle in the oesophagus.

Overbreathing (i.e. thoracic breathing pattern, thoracic respiration, abnormal breathing or hyperventilation) – A shallow pattern of thoracic breathing which can be associated with chest pain and breathlessness. If it causes movement of larger volumes of air in inspiration and expiration than normal, it will lead to hypocapnia (see previous).

Pacing – A skill taught in CBT that helps people to carry out activities regularly in a way that is sustainable and that avoids overexertion.

Peristalsis – The contractions of muscles within the digestive tract that move food along.

Psychoeducation – Providing psychologically based information to help a patient understand the processes involved in their chest pain (e.g. offering an explanation about the mechanisms of anxiety).

Rapid access chest pain clinic (RACPC) – A specialist clinic based in a hospital where GPs can refer patients with chest pain that could be of cardiac origin.

Safety-seeking behaviour – A type of coping strategy used to reduce anxiety that arises when a specific threat occurs but which leads to increased anxiety in the longer term.

Selective attention – Focusing on a specific object in one's environment (including physical sensations) whilst ignoring other information that may be occurring.

ST segment – The repolarisation wave of the ECG that is raised in myocardial infarction and depressed in ischaemia.

Index